Just the

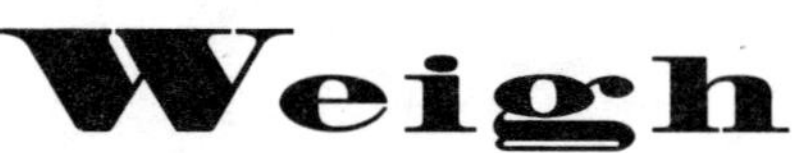

You Are

Just the Weigh You Are

How to Be Fit *and* Healthy, Whatever Your Size

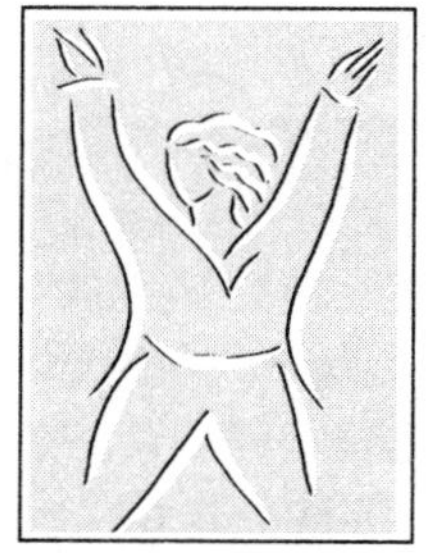

Steven Jonas, M.D.
and Linda Konner

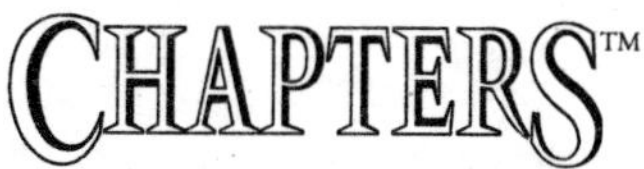

Chapters Publishing, Ltd., Shelburne, Vermont 05482

Published by
Chapters Publishing, Ltd.,
2085 Shelburne Road, Shelburne, VT 05482

Library of Congress Cataloging-in-Publication Data

Jonas, Steven.
Just the weigh you are: how to be fit and healthy, whatever your size / Steven Jonas, Linda Konner; illustrated by Paula Munck.
p. cm.
Includes index.
ISBN 1-57630-026-9
1. Overweight persons—Health and hygiene. 2. Overweight persons—Life skills guides. I. Konner, Linda. II. Title.
RA776.5.J5636 1997
613—DC21 96-39847

Printed and bound in Canada by
Webcom Limited, Scarborough, Ontario

Designed by Susan McClellan

Cover illustration by Paula Munck

For my mother.

—L.K.

To the memory of
Harold
and
Jeanne Jonas.

—S.J.

Acknowledgments

Special thanks to our excellent and always good-natured editor, Barry Estabrook, as well as to Gareth Esersky, a terrific agent and friend.

Contents

Authors' Note

Throughout this book, we use a variety of words and phrases interchangeably to identify the reader at whom this book is aimed. Those words and phrases include "overweight," "obese," "large," and "large-size." Obviously, because we take a pro-health, nondiet stance, the words and phrases used here are meant to be descriptive, not judgmental.

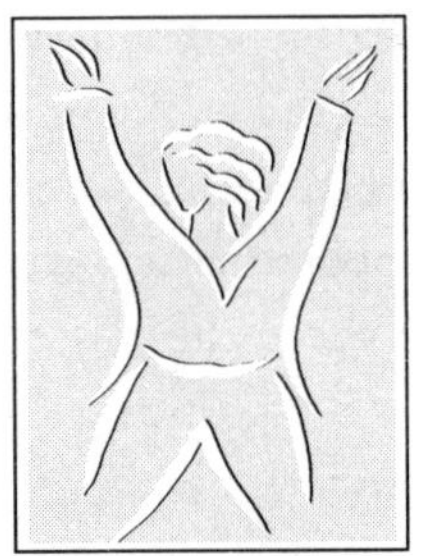

Wellness, Yes; Weight Loss, Not Necessarily

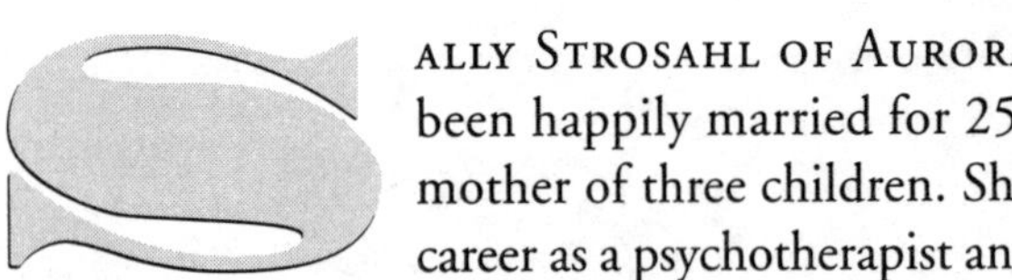

SALLY STROSAHL OF AURORA, ILLINOIS, has been happily married for 25 years and is the mother of three children. She has an exciting career as a psychotherapist and marriage counselor, and you might say she's something of a fitness nut—she eats healthy foods, she uses her NordicTrack several times a week, and she bikes in the summer and cross-country skis in the winter. Her blood pressure's normal, her cholesterol is low, and, generally speaking, she feels great.

Oh, did we mention that Sally weighs 260 pounds?

Something is happening in America in 1997, something big—in every sense of the word. For one thing, we Americans are getting heavier. According to the Centers for Disease Control and Prevention, one-fourth of all Americans were overweight in 1980; a decade later, that percentage climbed to one-third. A reanalysis of the data for 1991-94, using a new World Health Organization definition of "overweight," was presented at the 1996 annual meeting of the North American Association for the Study of Obesity. According to the latest analysis, more than *one-half* of adult Americans are overweight.

Not a great statistic, by any means, but there *is* a refreshing and very positive trend accompanying it. It seems that we, as a nation, are starting to get smarter about the entire issue of weight. We're not letting our weight get us as hung up as we once did. We want to look good, of course, but we're no longer willing to risk our health and our sanity for it. We're realizing that there's more to life than rigorously counting fat grams and wearing a size 8. We're starting to understand the implications of the statistic we've long heard, that just 5 to 10 percent of those who lose weight in an organized weight-loss program are able to keep it off permanently. We're accepting the fact that the only people around with bodies like Cindy Crawford's and Brad Pitt's are, well, Cindy Crawford and Brad Pitt. We're coming to terms, at long last, with who we are and what we weigh.

Just consider these facts:

• There are more organizations than ever acknowledging and accepting overweight people, including the 5,000-member National Association to Advance Fat Acceptance (with 50 branches nationwide), Abundia, and the National Association of Full-Figured Women. There is even a 300-member group of health professionals, called the Association of Health Enrichment of Large Persons (AHELP), to enable obesity experts to serve their overweight clients better without necessarily encouraging them to lose weight.

• For an increasing number of people, losing weight is far less a priority than it used to be. In a 1996 nationwide poll conducted for *Adweek* magazine, a whopping 82 percent said they'd rather be richer than slimmer. Even among those overweight individuals questioned, a healthy 76 percent came up with the same response.

• A growing number of men have "come out of the closet" and now proudly admit their affection for and attraction to Rubenesque women. One of them, Ken Mayer, the author of *Real Women Don't Diet*, showed that women could be overweight and at the same time feel sexy and desirable.

• More and more women are accepting the fact that they don't resemble the stick-thin Calvin Klein model Kate Moss—nor should they even try to. According to a spokeswoman for the fashion company Tahari Ltd., the typical sample size worn by models is a 6—while according to the May 8, 1996, *Wall Street Journal*, retailers report that more than one-third of American women actually wear a size 14 or larger.

• Thanks to groundbreaking books like Naomi Wolf's *The Beauty Myth*, more and more women have come to realize that they've been dieting for years for the wrong reasons and are finally freeing themselves from the pressure of trying to be skinny. Wolf outlined the ways in which advertisers, women's magazines, the media, and the manufacturers of diet-oriented products have jointly conspired to send the message that women can't be appealing unless they're thin, a state that's difficult or impossible for the majority of them to sustain. They're now rejecting these values and deciding to lose weight for themselves—or not at all.

• The nondiet approach to health has been under way for some time in Canada. A nationwide public-awareness campaign called Vitality, created by Health and Welfare Canada, deemphasizes body weight and encourages people to take charge of their health and the way they eat and to adopt a positive attitude about themselves, regardless of their size. And the 10-year-old Winnipeg-based group HUGS International, which was started by nutritionist Linda Omichinski and whose goal is to "free its members from the diet mentality and promote a normal, nondiet lifestyle," has 100 licensees in five countries.

• International No-Diet Day is an annual event, first celebrated on May 5, 1994, with the presentation by Alice Mahon, a member of the British Parliament, of this motion in the House of Commons: "This House supports National No-Diet Day . . . and notes that dieting undermines women's emotional and physical well-being . . . is concerned that dieting has reached epidemic levels . . . believes that the tyranny of thinness encourages women to be valued on their looks alone and encourages the oppression of fat people . . . and realizes that, while obesity may cause health risks to some people, the solution is not the simple answer of losing weight, because 96 percent of diets don't work . . ."

No question: There is a real diet backlash going on out there. Not only is the word "diet" seldom used anymore among health professionals, but more and more of them are coming to the realization that it's better to promote *health* and *weight maintenance*, whatever one's weight, than a weight-loss program that's likely to produce frustration and temporary results.

In the September/October 1992 issue of *Healthy Weight Journal*, editor Frances M. Berg, M.S., wrote: "A new movement is rising from the turmoil of widespread frustration with diets that don't work, pressures to be thin, and the crises in eating disorders that grip America. It calls for wellness, not weight loss, and it focuses on the following three factors: 1) feeling good about oneself; 2) eating well in a natural, relaxed way; and 3) being comfortably active."

We couldn't agree more, and this is precisely the approach we have taken in *Just the Weigh You Are.* Here, we hope to guide you toward maintaining *balance* in your life, based on setting and achieving a number of goals that may *not* include weighing what some standardized height-weight chart says you should weigh or what some skinny model makes you think you should weigh. Achieving that critical balance will, in turn, enable you to become healthier, whether or not you lose weight.

Our primary focus–and we feel strongly that it ought to be yours too—is on *health*, not weight. Recognizing that there are many factors besides body weight that affect health, we insist that you need not be condemned to a state of ill health—nor even *think* of yourself as unhealthy—for the rest of your life if you cannot or simply don't want to lose weight for any one of a number of perfectly legitimate physical, psychological, or social reasons. There are many other steps that you can take besides losing weight to improve your health and well-being. On the assumption that you'd like to live a long, healthy life, we'd like to show you how.

Just the Weigh You Are is, above all, a pro-health book. In fact, it may well be the first book co-written by a medical doctor who does not automatically recommend weight loss as the only path to better health for overweight people. Instead, what you'll find here is clear-cut evidence based on scientific research that proves overweight and wellness need not be mutually exclusive. You will quickly learn—regardless of what you may have believed up until now—that it's quite possible to lead a happy, active, fulfilling life whatever you weigh.

At the same time, *Just the Weigh You Are* is a pro-choice book. Unlike other "diet books" that spell out strict weight-loss plans for you to follow, or even other books dealing with self-acceptance, ours is not going to tell you what to do about your weight one way or the other. We want you to make up your own mind, and then, once *you* decide what you want to do, we'll outline the ways—comfortable, doable ways—to maximize the quality of your life.

In keeping with our basic philosophy, we will, for example, reinforce the importance of maintaining what is a *reasonable weight* for you—a concept quite different from the "ideal weight" or "healthy weight" you may have been unsuccessfully striving toward for years. Since reaching an aesthetic ideal or even a "healthy weight" as determined for you by someone else is impossible for many overweight people, the best course of action may simply be to aim for a weight that's easy for you to achieve and maintain. That weight may, in your particular case, be just 10 percent less than what you weigh now, or it may be your current weight. (We'll be showing you how to determine your reasonable weight in Chapter Two.)

And while this book does not necessarily advocate weight loss for large-size people, one of the mantras you're going to be hearing throughout these pages is "exercise." Sure, exercise is always touted as a key ingredient in weight loss, and it is. But even if you're not currently in a weight-reduction mode, you'll find that our exercise program—designed specifically for large-size women and men—will do wonders for both your physical *and* mental health, whether or not you wind up losing an ounce.

It is our aim to show you the Big Picture that is your life and to help you realize—despite everything you may have heard or read—that being healthy and feeling great is much, much more than a number on the scale or around your waist. There's so much we can do at *any* weight to reduce our health risks, increase our life expectancy and simply feel better and more energetic every day. Here, in the pages of *Just the Weigh You Are*, we will guide you, step by step, so that you can make those positive changes happen.

Chapter One

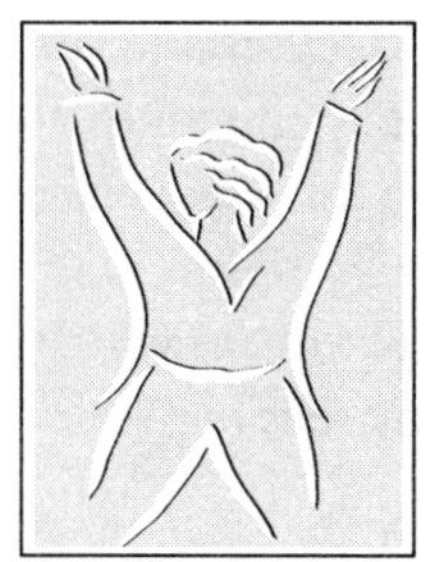

You May Stop Dieting Now

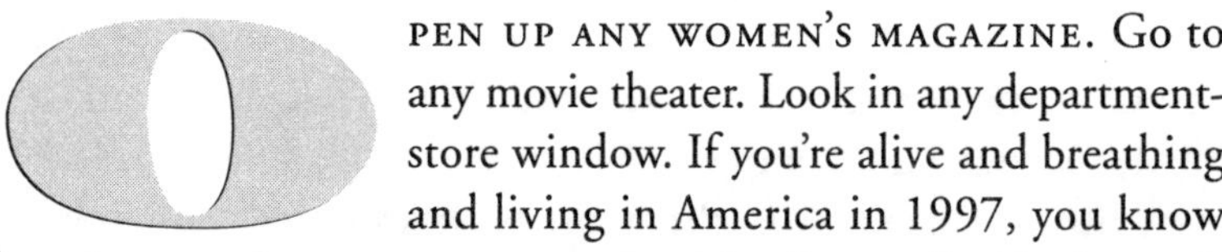

OPEN UP ANY WOMEN'S MAGAZINE. Go to any movie theater. Look in any department-store window. If you're alive and breathing and living in America in 1997, you know how intense the pressures are to be thin. Some of us lucky souls come by thinness naturally or with little effort. Others among us work like the devil to keep those extra pounds as far from our thighs and bellies as possible.

But many of us—most of us, in fact—have real-life bodies that are not going to be appearing in a Calvin Klein underwear ad any-time soon. Still, while that is indeed the reality, reality can be hard to accept when we grow up conditioned to believe that Thin Is In, that Slim Is Better Than Fat. Even if we're blessed with an essentially healthy, strong sense of ourselves that tells us we're fine, worth-while people regardless of our 42-inch hips, there's a warring side of us that somehow doesn't believe it. It's the voice that whispers into our brain daily—every time we reach for that bread basket, every time we decide to sleep in instead of go to the gym—that we're *not* so good after all. We're not as thin as Oprah has become. We can't fit into the same size jeans Mel Gibson can. What's *wrong* with us?

The answer is: nothing. For despite how long you may have believed otherwise, **you are not your weight.** Your weight is merely one part of who you are, how you look, how you feel—and how healthy you might be. To equate your *self* with a number on the scale is not something any sensible person should be doing. What's more, it isn't necessary.

This is one of the few places anywhere you're going to hear the following true statement: You can be relatively healthy and feel good about yourself, too, regardless of your weight. And we're going to show you how. So if you've never before given yourself permission to finally stop dieting for weight loss, we are officially granting you that permission, right now.

Why are we doing this? Because we know how frustrating, often futile, and potentially harmful weight-loss/weight-maintenance efforts are for many people. Both of us have been there personally, and we've also worked with hundreds of thousands of people—through our books and magazine articles and in one-on-one sessions—whose repeated attempts to shed pounds and keep them off have made them unhappy, angry, and often heavier than they were when they began. Furthermore, the statistics back up the commonly accepted beliefs that, for many of us, weight loss is temporary, and dieting frequently starts a cycle that ends with our adding, not subtracting, pounds.

Now, we're not saying here that obesity is a good thing. In fact, a 16-year study conducted on 115,000 nurses, published in the September 14, 1995, issue of *The New England Journal of Medicine*, concluded that even a moderate weight gain—as little as 18 pounds—put otherwise-healthy women at increased risk for heart disease, cardiovascular death, and cancer. Yes, overweight *is* a risk factor for ill health. (There'll be a greater discussion of risk factors in Chapter Two.) If you are one of those people who are able to lose weight and keep it off, congratulations and more power to you. But, as we have said and as you well know, many overweight people simply cannot, for one reason or another, do that successfully. If such is the case for you, we are here to happily tell you that you needn't think that you are condemned to a lifetime of poor health, because weight is only *one* factor in determining overall health.

Let's repeat that important thought, because it's central to the theme of this book: *Your weight is only one of the factors that determine your overall health.* There are many others—how and what you eat (there are healthy and unhealthy eating habits, whether you lose weight or not); whether you exercise (yes, overweight people can and should exercise, whether they lose weight or not); whether you smoke cigarettes; whether you use other drugs such as alcohol in a healthy or unhealthy way; whether you can successfully manage stress; and so forth. In this book, we are going to show you how, if you are overweight, you can still lead a happy, healthy life by getting those other, easier-to-handle risk factors under control.

Okay, We're Overweight. So How'd We Get This Way in the First Place?

IT'S AN AWFULLY GOOD THING that weight isn't the sole determinant of health because, despite our national obsession with thinness, it remains an elusive dream for millions of us. Why? Several reasons. First, we live in a society that encourages weight gain:

• the proliferation of fast-food places with their high-fat offerings;

• our get-it-done-now lifestyles, which lead to overeating because of career pressures and other stresses;

• two-job households, which often mean unstructured eating routines and the development of poor eating habits by all members of the family;

• a mind-boggling array of labor-saving devices, everything from push-button car-window openers to electric pencil sharpeners, all discouraging even the slightest physical activity.

Those are just four of the likely environmental causes.

Many of us who are overweight have practiced the art of eating too much and exercising too little for a long time. Let's face it: In this society of ours, eating excessive quantities of the wrong kinds of food and neglecting exercise is easy. Poor eating habits are shockingly simple to develop and sustain, whether they begin in childhood, with pregnancy, following the loss of a loved one, or during a career crisis. In this part of the world, fattening food is plentiful—and inexpensive. For just pennies, we can "supersize" our already fat-packed meal, and doughnuts are usually cheaper by the dozen.

But there is another reason why people who become overweight just once, as adults, have a very hard time ever getting thin again: our national obsession with dieting. Even with a concerted effort to start eating the vegetables and hitting that StairMaster every day, weight loss may be difficult or impossible. If you're a yo-yo dieter from way back, that constant adding and subtracting of fat from your body may have permanently changed your metabolism—specifically, it may have lowered your resting metabolic rate (RMR), the rate at which your body uses calories when you're inactive.

To explain: Whenever you lose weight, you lose some fat (which is good) and some lean muscle mass (which is not so good, because muscle mass is what helps keep your body a lean, mean, fat-burning machine). But whenever you *regain* weight as a result of overeating, you add only fat, because now you're taking in too many calories in relationship to the needs of your body, and it will automatically store many of those calories as body fat. With all that extra stored fat and proportionately less muscle, your body becomes less metabolically efficient than it was before, and so it takes more work than ever to burn the calories you consume. Some people may be able to raise their RMR by building up muscle mass through a regular program of aerobic and weight-training exercise—but, unfortunately, many won't.

Another way your RMR may have been adversely affected is by the little-discussed but scientifically established phenomenon known as diet-induced low-calorie overweight (LCO). How can you be overweight if you're eating a low-calorie diet? The explanation hails from the days of our hunter-gatherer ancestors, who knew that finding food was frequently iffy at best. Luckily for them, their bodies could adapt to a possible drop-off in the wild-turkey or elderberry supply in one of two ways: 1) by storing excess food eaten during times of plenty as body fat, to be used later on as energy; and 2) by lowering their RMR. This second response is known as the "starvation response," and it kept cavefolks from wasting away until the local ShopRite could restock wild-turkey burgers. What would happen was that, once their bodies sensed that food might not be available for a while, their highly flexible metabolisms reacted by slowing down significantly to be able to use the available edibles more efficiently, thus preserving both life and limb until the food supply returned to normal. By lowering the RMR, the body could, with any luck, accomplish this while keeping body weight stable.

Today, in the 1990s, the starvation response is alive and well whenever you deliberately attempt to starve yourself by suddenly going on a very-low-calorie diet. Let's say you want to drop some pounds, and to try to do that, one day you start eating the latest "miracle" 900-calorie-a-day diet, which is fairly close to starving yourself. Your body, used to getting its usual supply of food, suddenly reacts like a caveman's body would, by saying, in effect, "Darn—out of wild-turkey burgers *again*! Better start slowing things down." So, believing it's being starved, your body responds by dropping the RMR.

The first couple of times you go on this type of calorie-slashing diet, you probably *will* lose weight, because your body's starvation response hasn't knocked your RMR down too much. But go on and off such diets enough times in your life, and you will depress your RMR to the point where you may never again be able to lose weight. And each time you "finish" such a diet, if you go back to anything like your pre-diet eating habits—that is, if the weight-loss program has taught you nothing about healthy, sensible eating—the weight lost will come right back, now that your calorie intake is up and your RMR is down. Once the RMR declines as a result of the starvation response, it doesn't come back up by itself. Your body has no way of reading the new signal, the one that says, "Diet's over." Once your body interprets the message as "Famine's coming," it has no way to know that it really *isn't.* Your RMR stays down—and your weight goes up.

But maybe the reason for *your* weight gain is different. You might have inherited some of those nasty "obesity genes" we've heard so much about, the ones said to biologically predispose some of us to overweight. Well, maybe. The existence of such a gene has been speculated about for decades, and while it apparently does exist, it would still not account for the sudden fat explosion, in this country alone, over the past 15 years or so.

For some people, overweight does have a genetic basis, which makes it especially hard for them to lose weight. However, the fact is, we're living through nothing less than an American obesity epidemic. We're getting very heavy at a very fast rate—much too fast for it to simply be attributed to an "obesity gene," because if indeed there is such a gene, this obesity epidemic should be cropping up in other countries as much as it is in ours. But it isn't. Therefore, any "obesity gene" might explain why some of us are overweight, but it doesn't explain why so many of us are, and so suddenly.

Oh, there are other reasons accounting for overweight. You may simply be unable to mobilize sufficient motivation to embark on a permanent weight-loss program, even though you might want to. Low-level motivation is very understandable—particularly if you've been frustrated in your efforts to lose weight in the past. (We will talk about motivation-mobilizing steps in Chapter Four.) Being overweight may also stem from one's fears of intimacy (of getting too close, figuratively *and* literally, to others), including the fear of one's own sexuality (as a large-size person, you will automatically be less sexually desirable to some part of the population).

Keep in mind that while we have a pretty good handle on the myriad causes of overweight, we still don't know how these various causes are distributed in the overweight population. Incredibly, nobody has ever done a broad-based study of the epidemiology of weight gain—that is, the characteristics of various groups of overweight people and the different factors associated with those groups. The explanations we've offered above account for most of the obesity in our population, but we can only guess at how many overweight people fall into each of the major groups or may have two different causes at work simultaneously.

Clearly, though, for a lot of us, weight is not just a result of calories in and calories out, as we've been taught to believe. There's much more going on—and the bottom line for many people is that, for all their genuine efforts, the weight is just not coming off.

Being Fat in Thin-Obsessed America

As we said at the outset, even with our country's increasingly obese population, there is nevertheless the constant pressure on us—especially on women—to be thin. On television, in movies, and in fashion magazines, thin men and women are held up as models of glamour and sex appeal. (Does any woman on "Melrose Place" wear anything larger than a size 4 dress?) Celebrities who have the money (to hire personal trainers to motivate them and chefs to prepare low-fat meals) and the time (to work out several hours per day) are meant to motivate those of us who have to work 10- and 12-hour days and have to cook our own meat loaf. We may have to eat like Roseanne, but we're told that we should be looking like Julia Roberts. Such a contradiction between what is and what many of us wish for, bodywise, has helped to feed our current $35 billion weight-loss industry. This weight-loss battle we're collectively fighting is a losing battle—but, unfortunately, not in the sense we'd like it to be.

When you combine the difficulty of weight loss/weight maintenance with society's pressures on us to be thin, what results is confusion, frustration, anger—and a segment of the population that's attacked on all fronts. If you're overweight, you're told, first and foremost, that your body is unattractive. Next, you're told you're weak—if you can't lose weight, it's your own fault, because anybody who truly wants to do it can. So you're inadequate and inept. And, as if all that weren't bad enough, you're told you're harming your body—that old if-you're-overweight-you-can't-possibly-be-healthy message. Regardless of anything else you might do to safeguard your health, goes the thinking, you're doomed to ill health because of your weight.

We are here to bring you a different message. As we have said before and will say again, *while significant overweight is not good for your health, if you are overweight and simply cannot lose for one reason or another, you should not feel that you are condemned to a life of ill health.* There are many other steps you can take to improve your life and longevity without losing weight.

And while it's easier said than done, we urge you to stop feeling unworthy because of your dress or pants size. Yes, you may be clear-eyed about what you eat every day and have good, perfectly justifiable reasons why you don't weigh 125 pounds. Although we're not going to let you off the hook completely and say that your present weight isn't at least *partly* your responsibility, we are going to tell you to stop blaming yourself for what you look like today. And even if you are "to blame," there may well be very sound reasons—metabolic, genetic, physiological, psychological—why you can't get thinner. After the lifelong conditioning you may have received, you may make poor food choices. Or you eat for emotional reasons that are now ingrained. Or you have always avoided exercise. You've got to stop, once and for all, kicking yourself for habits that may have been established over a period of 10, 20, 30 or more years. Before you became heavy, you may not have been taught that the key to staying at your normal body weight is healthy eating and exercise. You may know it now, but that information may have come along too late for you to be able to radically alter your body shape and size.

Also, as we said earlier, you may not be motivated right now to embark on the full-fledged lifestyle change necessary for lifelong weight control—even if it's physiologically possible for you. If that's the case, you should wait until you are really ready, rather than make another half-hearted attempt at weight loss. One reason some people can't lose weight is that they can't mobilize their motivation sufficiently to complete the job. That's legitimate, and it's no less valid an explanation than saying you're overweight for genetic reasons or because your body size is the result of low-calorie overweight. And it *certainly* doesn't make you a bad person. Simply accept your decision without judgment. Maybe a year from now, maybe a month from now, you'll feel differently. But for now, this is how it is.

Of course, if you *are* genuinely motivated to launch a serious weight-loss program, we'd be the last ones to try to stop you. But we understand how difficult weight-loss motivation can be to find and hold on to, particularly after repeated attempts have failed. So . . . lose the guilt and the bad feelings. Recognize that you can become healthier without losing weight. Get on with the business of doing just that.

Read on, and we'll start showing you how.

Top Ten Reasons to Give Up Dieting

#10: Diets don't work. Even if you lose weight, you will probably gain it all back, and you might gain back more than you lost.

#9: Diets are expensive. If you didn't buy special diet products, you could save enough to get new clothes, which would improve your outlook right now.

#8: Diets are boring. People on diets talk and think about food and practically nothing else. There's a lot more to life.

#7: Diets don't necessarily improve your health. Like the weight loss, the health improvement is temporary. Dieting can actually cause health problems.

#6: Diets don't make you beautiful. Very few people will ever look like models. Glamour is a look, not a size. You don't have to be thin to be attractive.

#5: Diets are not sexy. If you want to be more attractive, take care of your body and your appearance. Feeling healthy makes you look your best.

#4: Diets can turn into eating disorders. The obsession to be thin can lead to anorexia, bulimia, bingeing, and compulsive exercising.

#3: Diets can make you afraid of food. Food nourishes and comforts us and gives us pleasure. Dieting can make food seem like your enemy and can deprive you of all the positive things about food.

#2: Diets can rob you of energy. If you want to lead a full and active life, you need good nutrition and enough food to meet your body's needs.

AND THE NUMBER ONE REASON TO GIVE UP DIETING . . .

#1: Learning to love and accept yourself just as you are will give you self-confidence, better health, and a sense of well-being that will last a lifetime.

PROFILE

Katie Arons

Los Angeles, California
Age: 30
Height: 5'10"
Weight: 230 to 240 pounds
Occupation: Model

I COME FROM A BIG FAMILY, in every sense of the word. I have five older brothers, and everybody is huge. My biggest brother is 6'5" and around 270 pounds. As for me, I was one of the biggest girls in school—in high school, I wore a size 24. It was very hard, and kids would make fun of me. I remember praying every night, "Please, God, please help me lose weight!"

Naturally, my family was very concerned about my weight, and I went on my first diet when I was 9. I continued trying to lose weight, going on and off every possible diet, until age 24. That's when I went to an endocrinologist and got my body chemistry straightened out—it got out of whack from crazy dieting all my life. The first thing the endocrinologist did was to put me on Optifast. For three months, I fasted. I didn't have a single bite of solid food, not even a celery stick or a cracker; I just drank the protein shakes. I was one of 15 people on this program, and I was the only one who didn't cheat. (You can't say that I have a problem with willpower!)

The first three weeks were torture, sheer hell, to the point where I tried to sleep as much as possible just so I wouldn't think about food. Then it got easier, and gradually the doctor took me off the shakes and "energy food" and put me on real food—plain, simply prepared meals. That was when I learned to appreciate things like steamed vegetables without salt and

PROFILE

butter. I still eat pretty well today—I'm basically a vegetarian. When I started on Optifast, I weighed 275 pounds, and after six months, including the three-month fast, I got down to 190. I was a size 12, and I stayed under 200 pounds for about six months. Then I leveled off at about 220 pounds—a size 16 or 18—and I was able to maintain that weight effortlessly, without dieting.

I was working at a hotel in Miami Beach when a scout for Ford Models approached me about doing some large-size modeling. I said yes immediately! My new, glamorous career was very exciting, especially after so many years of feeling bad about my body, but something was wrong. For some reason, my weight was suddenly creeping back up. I didn't understand what was going on.

Then, one day, I reached a turning point. I had been modeling for about a year and a half, and I was in New York on a photo shoot for *Big Beautiful Woman* magazine. One of the editors at the shoot came over to me and said, "You know, Katie, we think you're beautiful, and we love your pictures. But there's something in your eyes that says you're not happy with yourself. My guess is that it's about your weight. You really need to do one of two things: either do something about your weight . . . or learn to accept yourself as you are."

I went home after the shoot, and I gave a lot of thought to what the editor had said. I thought about my life at that time, when I weighed 230 pounds, and how it compared with the way it was when I weighed 190. The fact was, there wasn't much of a difference. I was always fantasizing about how nice it would be to be back at 190 pounds, but in order to do that, I knew I'd have to start dieting again. That meant I'd have to start worrying about my weight, what I ate, and all of that all over again. At 230 pounds, I didn't have those worries. True, I had moved up a couple of dress sizes, but I could still wear

PROFILE

nice clothes. I was very healthy—I rarely got sick, and I could pretty much do everything my friends did. I had a good career—I was one of the most successful large-size print models in the country. I dated nice guys. Best of all, I had to admit that at the higher weight, I felt much freer—it was such a relief not to have to worry about whether what I was eating was against the diet "rules." It was great to live without guilt.

That's when I decided to stop dieting forever. It took me a long time to get to that point, but I'm much happier, and I want to share these feelings so that I can help other people feel better about themselves. I get especially upset by young girls who are obsessed with dieting because they're not bone-thin. It's such a waste of time; there are so many better things you can do with your life. I'm often asked to be a commentator at fashion shows, and I love the fact that it enables me to talk to lots of young girls and be a positive role model for them.

I'll never forget how once, after a fashion show, the mother of a 12-year-old girl came up to me. Her daughter had been in the audience, and as one of the biggest girls in her school, the girl had always felt bad about her weight. But after hearing my comments about self-acceptance, she said, "Mom, I think I'm going to be okay." I thought that was wonderful. Young girls don't get this message nearly enough, the message that it's okay to weigh what you weigh and to accept yourself. But I'm going to get on my soapbox and send out the word every chance I get!

CHAPTER TWO

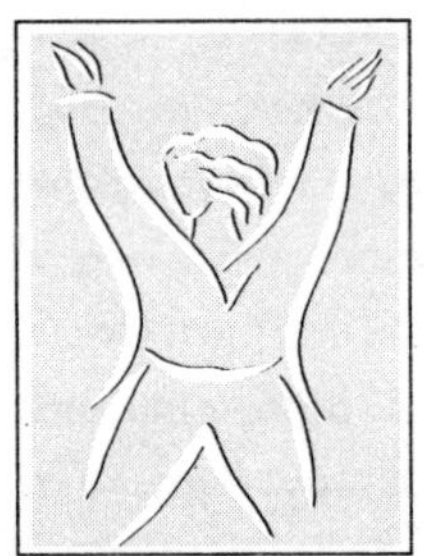

Weight, Fat, and Your Health Risks

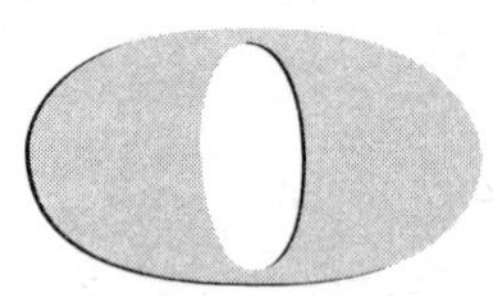

OVERWEIGHT EQUALS ILLNESS, RIGHT? Not so fast. We've been hearing reports for decades that excess pounds bring with them a vast array of health problems, not to mention a decreased life expectancy. In fact, that frightening message has been hammered into our heads so much and for so long that most of us believe it unquestioningly. But we think it's time we all questioned this assumption.

It is true that many reputable studies have been done over the years conclusively linking obesity to such conditions as adult-onset (Type II) diabetes, hypertension, joint disease (especially of the knees), increased serum-cholesterol level, and gallbladder disease. Obesity is frequently a precursor of heart disease, and it's possible that it may lead directly to heart disease as well as to certain types of cancer, such as cancer of the breast and/or colon.

Yes, excess weight increases the risk of ill health and can lead to extra trips to the doctor's office. For some segment of the population (including you, perhaps), weight reduction is a very good idea if it results in more manageable diabetes, for example, or a better blood-pressure reading. If that's the case, we strongly encourage you to try to lose some weight in order to improve your present level of health. Later in this book (Chapter Five), we'll outline the best, most sensible ways to go about it.

However, it may be that you are already one of those folks who are overweight and disease-free, someone who, on a day-to-day basis, feels just fine—healthy, active, and generally unencumbered by your size. If you fit that description, you know that sweeping generalizations about the overweight/ill-health connection just don't ring true. What's more, you're far from alone. There are plenty of folks out there whose weight may be an occasional hassle but who otherwise feel good and capable of doing pretty much whatever they want to do. The stories of many such women and men are scattered throughout the pages of this book. They easily dispel the myth that you can't be heavy and healthy at the same time.

What Is Overweight? What Is Overfat?

And How Do These States Affect Your Health?

REGARDLESS OF HOW GOOD you may be feeling, it's important to know where your particular body size fits into the whole health picture and whether your weight is or is not jeopardizing your well-being. But how will you know if you don't understand the various terms used in books and magazine articles and by doctors? To help clarify the matter, we offer the following mini glossary.

Obese (or Overfat): A state of having too much body fat (see Table 1, page 32). In most cases, an obese person (that is, one who carries excess body fat) is also an overweight person (who carries an excess number of pounds), but not necessarily. One can be of normal weight and obese at the same time.

Overweight: A body weight that is anything above the established normal range for your gender, height and age (see Table 2, opposite).

Minimal overweight: A weight that is 1 to 20 percent above the upper end of the established normal weight range for your gender, height, and age (see Table 2). This weight range carries no known health risks.

Mild overweight: A body weight that is 21 to 40 percent above the upper end of the established normal weight range for your gender, height, and age. This weight range does not seem to carry perceptible health risks, but might.

Moderate overweight: A body weight that is 41 to 100 percent above the upper end of the established normal weight range for your gender, height, and age. Health risks seem to increase at this weight range.

Morbid (or severe) overweight: A body weight that is 101 percent or more above the upper end of the established normal weight range for your gender, height, and age. Morbid obesity places you at serious health risk and may decrease longevity.

Table 1: Percentages of Body Fat

	Women	Men
Athletes	less than 17% body fat	less than 10% body fat
Lean	17-22%	10-15%
Normal	22-25%	15-18%
Above average	25-29%	18-20%
Overfat	29-35%	20-25%
Obese	35-plus%	25-plus%

Table 2: Are You Overweight?

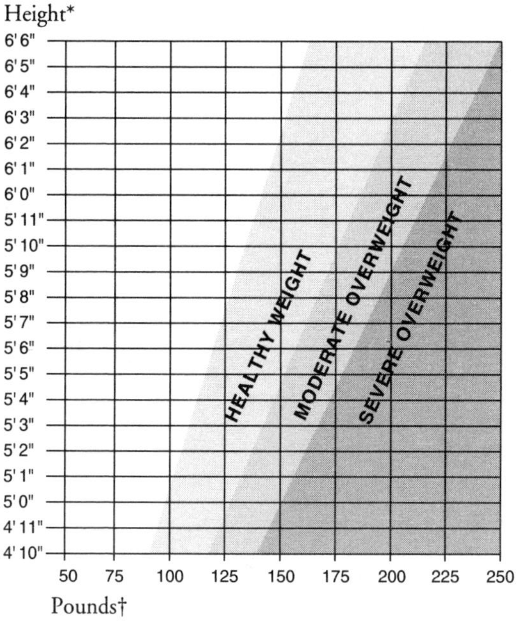

Height*

6'6"
6'5"
6'4"
6'3"
6'2"
6'1"
6'0"
5'11"
5'10"
5'9"
5'8"
5'7"
5'6"
5'5"
5'4"
5'3"
5'2"
5'1"
5'0"
4'11"
4'10"

HEALTHY WEIGHT
MODERATE OVERWEIGHT
SEVERE OVERWEIGHT

50 75 100 125 150 175 200 225 250

Pounds†

*Without shoes.

†Without clothes. The higher weights apply to people with more muscle and bone, such as many men.

From the 1995 Report of the Dietary Guidelines Advisory Committee on the Dietary Guidelines for Americans

How Useful Is Knowing Your Weight?

When a person talks about her body size, she usually describes it using the standard measurement used in this country: weight in pounds, that number that glares up at you from your bathroom scale every Monday morning. But the fact is, that number isn't always helpful, and it doesn't necessarily give you the most accurate information about your body's state of health. Remember that a scale measures not only the fat in your body but also critical components such as fluids (water and blood), bone, and muscle. So indeed, you might go "off the chart" on a typical height/weight table if you were to focus solely on your weight, yet you might, in fact, be the picture of health.

For instance, let's say you're a 31-year-old woman who's 5'10" and weighs 180 pounds. By most standardized charts, you'd be regarded as overweight. Yet you might be a well-conditioned runner who takes part in marathons regularly and who has just 15 percent body fat. Should you go on a weight-reducing diet? You might be tempted to if you swore by the charts—as, regrettably, so many people do. But it might not be advisable—or necessary. Just as the scale is able to give you just one small piece of information about yourself, your weight is able to give you just one small piece of information about your state of health.

Measuring Body Fat

A RELATIVELY NEW TOOL being used by doctors and others concerned with our weight is the Body Mass Index, or BMI. (Its use is the basis for the 1996 finding cited in the Introduction that more than half of adult Americans are overweight.) Your BMI is found by multiplying your weight in pounds by 700, dividing that number by your height in inches, then dividing again by your height in inches, but all the math has been done for you in the BMI chart (Table 3, opposite).

At first glance, it may seem as though this table is just a fancy height/weight chart. In fact, unlike some height/weight charts you may have been using, this one does not take into account factors such as age or sex. But because the BMI *does* figure your body-fat percentage into the equation, not just your weight—and because percentage of body fat is considered a more accurate gauge of health than weight in pounds—many experts use the BMI to help them assess health risks. Numbers higher than 27 on the BMI represent a body-fat proportion in excess of 30 percent for women and 25 percent for men, levels that may contribute to the usual obesity-

Table 3: Body Mass Index (BMI)

Height (inches)	19	20	21	22	23	24	25	26	27	28	29	30	35	40
							Body Weight (pounds)							
58	91	96	100	105	110	115	119	124	129	134	138	143	167	191
59	94	99	104	109	114	119	124	128	133	138	143	148	173	198
60	97	102	107	112	118	123	128	133	138	143	148	153	179	204
61	100	106	111	116	122	127	132	137	143	148	153	158	185	211
62	104	109	115	120	126	131	136	142	147	153	158	164	191	218
63	107	113	118	124	130	135	141	146	152	158	163	169	197	225
64	110	116	122	128	134	140	145	151	157	163	169	174	204	232
65	114	120	126	132	138	144	150	156	162	168	174	180	210	240
66	118	124	130	136	142	148	155	161	167	173	179	186	216	247
67	121	127	134	140	146	153	159	166	172	178	185	191	223	255
68	125	131	138	144	151	158	164	171	177	184	190	197	230	262
69	128	135	142	149	155	162	169	176	182	189	196	203	236	270
70	132	139	146	153	160	167	174	181	188	195	202	207	243	278
71	136	143	150	157	165	172	179	186	193	200	208	215	250	286
72	140	147	154	162	169	177	184	191	199	206	213	221	258	294
73	144	151	159	166	174	182	189	197	204	212	219	227	265	302
74	148	155	163	171	179	186	194	202	210	218	225	233	272	311
75	152	160	168	176	184	192	200	208	216	224	232	240	279	319
76	156	164	172	180	189	197	205	213	221	230	238	246	287	328

To use the table, find the appropriate height in the left-hand column. Move across to a given weight. The boldface number at the top of the column is the Body Mass Index at that height and weight.

Interpreting Your BMI Number

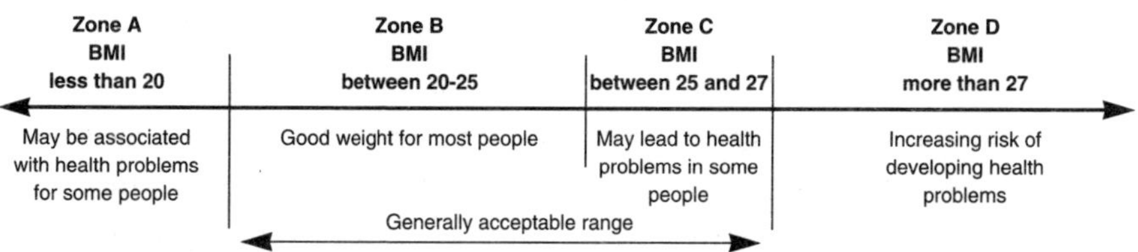

From Obesity & Health, Sept./Oct. 1993

related health risks: heart disease, hypertension and stroke, Type II diabetes, certain types of cancer, and gallbladder disease.

Some obesity experts are now using another formula to assess whether your body-fat percentage is jeopardizing health—the waist-hip ratio, or WHR—based on the idea that your waist measurement is a good indication of your health risk. To compute your WHR, measure your waist at the narrowest point between the bottom of your rib cage and the top of your pelvis. Then divide that number by the size of your hips (in inches) at the widest protrusion of your buttocks. The resulting number is your WHR. A WHR higher than 0.8 for a woman or 1.0 for a man indicates that you're carrying more abdominal fat than is good for your health. A variation on this theme uses a simple tape measure to get similar results. It is felt that a woman with a waist measurement of 31" should not gain any more weight, and she should definitely lose weight for health reasons if her current waist measurement is 34" or higher. Similarly, a man with a waist measurement over 37" is at his top weight for health considerations, and if his waist is 40" or above, he would be well advised to go on a weight-reduction program.

This method of correlating health risk to waist measurement ties in to the widely held belief that health risk is as much determined by where our body fat is located as it is by the *amount* of body fat we carry. In general, it appears to be riskier for anyone to carry excess fat around the midsection than elsewhere. One reason for this may be that when located in that area, excess fat is likelier to interfere with the normal functioning of major body organs. Women tend to accumulate their excess body fat around their hips and thighs, producing something of a pear-shaped body, while overweight men are more inclined to be "apple-shaped," gathering excess fat around the stomach (sometimes lovingly known as a beer belly). One key exception to this tendency occurs when women reach menopause, when hormonal changes cause the fat to shift upward from their lower regions to their stomach area, giving them a more squarish, boxy figure and placing them at a health risk very similar to their potbellied brothers and husbands. If you and/or your doctor feel that the location of your body fat may put you at excessive health risk, then you might want to consider losing some weight overall through a sensible food plan and regular exercise.

A Final Word on Standardized Measures

When it comes to *your* weight and *your* health, there are no absolutes that you can read off a chart, no matter how authoritative that chart may appear to be. You must always remember that height/weight charts, body-fat percentage tables and other measuring formulas—even the ones you see in this book—reflect *averages* determined from *groups* of people. These facts and figures help life-insurance companies, doctors, nutritionists, athletic trainers, and others in the health-care business (and you, too) know what the national averages are. But they don't necessarily tell you as an *individual*, someone who may want to improve his or her health, exactly what you need to do. Everybody—and every body—is different and must be judged on an individual basis.

It's the *balance* of factors that determines your health, how you feel, and how you feel about yourself, not any one factor standing alone. That's why it's silly to get too hung up about trying to conform to a particular set of weight "requirements"—*and* why it's critical for you to take responsibility for as much of your health care as you can.

What's best for *your* body and what *you* can do for it may be different from someone else's best. If you're not feeling as well as you could be and want to be and you're overweight, consider the possibilities. Maybe it's your weight—but maybe it's not.

What Is Health, Anyway?

YOU MAY DEFINE "HEALTH" as anything from being able to climb Mount Kilimanjaro to being able to climb out of bed in the morning—it's that personal. In this book, we use a definition of health based on the one developed by the World Health Organization and several other respected authorities:

"A state of well-being, of feeling good about oneself, of optimum functioning, of the absence of disease, and of the control and reduction of both internal and external risk factors for both disease and negative health conditions."

When we are talking about weight, as in this book, the key element of this definition is the term "risk factor." It can be defined as some environmental element, personal habit, or living condition that increases the likelihood of developing, at some time in the future, a particular disease or negative health condition. Within the context of weight-related problems, diabetes and cancer are examples of diseases, while elevated serum cholesterol is a negative health condition, and hypertension can be regarded as either a risk factor *or* a disease. Among the risk factors for obesity are overeating, a sedentary lifestyle, sudden calorie-restriction dieting, genetic predisposition, unmanaged stress, and excess alcoholic-beverage consumption, especially of beer.

Personal Health Checklist

YOUR DOCTOR OR OTHER HEALTH-CARE professional may tell you that you need to lose weight. The latest newspaper article on obesity and its outcomes may suggest that you need to lose weight. Even your loving mother may be urging you to drop a few pounds. But *should* you even try on the assumption that it will improve your health? Answering the following 10 questions will give you a good idea of the current state of your health and whether or not your weight poses a special health risk *for you:*

1. I have been diagnosed as having high blood pressure.
Yes_____ No_____

2. I have been diagnosed as having cardiovascular disease.
Yes_____ No_____

3. I have been diagnosed as having diabetes.
Yes_____ No_____

4. I have a history of breathing problems, although I do not smoke.
Yes_____ No_____

5. I use prescription medication on a regular basis.
Yes_____ No_____

6. I suffer from bone and/or joint problems.
Yes_____ No_____

7. My energy level is very low/I'm tired much of the time.
Yes_____ No_____

8. I experience sleep difficulties.
Yes_____ No_____

9. My sex drive is low or nonexistent.
Yes_____ No_____

10. I have little or no zest for living.
Yes_____ No_____

Using this checklist is not, of course, the same as going to your doctor for a complete, up-to-date health-status evaluation. (And, needless to say, if the answers to these questions seem to reveal a serious problem, you should by all means discuss your concerns with your health-care professional as soon as possible.) However, this information should give you a pretty clear picture of your current state of health. The disease and negative health conditions listed above are sometimes the result of, or may be made worse by, overweight.

Even if you checked Yes to only one or two of the questions above, your condition may be improved by weight loss, even a small one. For example, diabetes risk is often reduced when an overweight person loses as little as 7 or 10 percent of her weight, and high blood pressure may disappear.

So, while losing weight might indeed help you if you're currently suffering from one or more of the above conditions, you need not be alarmed if you can't or don't choose to lose weight. You can still, in many cases, improve your health with an alternate plan of action, which we'll be outlining in upcoming chapters.

Time to Get Real

SO OFTEN PEOPLE ASK US, "Steve, what should someone like me who's 5'5" weigh?" or, "Linda, do you agree with the latest study that says it's bad for your health if you're more than X percent overweight?"

We're eager to be of help, but there are two different kinds of answers we can give. First, we can give specific answers like these: The *average* person who is 5'5" tall is described as having a "healthy weight" if he or she is in the 115-to-150-pound range; and, yes, for the *population as a whole*, overweight above a certain level is a definite risk factor for certain diseases. But for someone struggling with a chronic, possibly lifelong weight problem, though, the answers may be quite different. They must be tailored to the individual's particular situation.

Obesity is no one's first choice. We've already acknowledged that there is sufficient documentation to implicate obesity in a number of chronic, life-shortening diseases. It *is* more likely than not that overweight people will have less external energy because of the internal energy they must expend to carry their weight around. Many overweight people frequently complain that they're more tired than they were when they were thinner, or than their thinner friends seem to be. And it's not uncommon for obese people to complain about ailments ranging from sleep apnea to painful joints, from breathing difficulties to low sex drive.

These problems aren't mythical, and despite our nondiet position, we want to make one point clear: We do not say that being overweight is a good thing. We do not deny that weight-related health woes and risks are very real for many people. You've been hearing about them—and perhaps living with them—for years, and for many folks, they are a fact of daily life. We'd be the first to say, Wouldn't it be nice if we could all lose weight to improve these conditions just like that, just by deciding to do so? National and personal medical bills would be slashed, we'd probably live a few years longer, and we'd feel better more of the time.

But let's get real. For reasons we've mentioned earlier—genetic overweight, the adverse effects of chronic dieting, motivation that has yet to be mobilized, and others—these weight-loss wishes may never come true. But, we're saying, don't throw in the towel. Weight is just one factor in determining health, and if you simply can't lose for one good reason or another, there are still many things you can do to improve your health and the way you feel. Furthermore, recent research has shown that except for morbid obesity, it may not be the weight that's the culprit here, but the sedentary (couch-potato) lifestyle that usually accompanies overweight.

It happens that the day-to-day health improvements you may make as a large-size person may actually result in more significant health improvements than if they were made by someone who's slim(mer). For example, if a sedentary, overweight person were to start exercising on a regular basis, she may not lose weight, but her health would likely improve in many ways—for example, increased energy levels, reduced stress, more restful sleep, and possibly the desire to eat more healthfully. That one behavior change—following a regular program of exercise—might actually help a large-size person proportionately more than it would a thinner person.

Current research supports the notion that, even if you remain overweight, working out and becoming fit can help you live longer. In one study done at the Cooper Institute for Aerobics Research, in Dallas, more than 25,000 obese men were given an initial health exam that included a treadmill test and a body-fat assessment. Eight years later, they were retested, and the men who were moderately fit or very fit had a 70 percent lower mortality rate than unfit men, after factors such as age, smoking habits, cholesterol levels, and overall health were taken into account. Mortality rates, it was concluded, were more influenced by the men's fitness levels than by their weight.

Furthermore, keep in mind that weight reduction is not an all-or-nothing issue, and if you are sufficiently motivated to drop some weight, we have good news: your "ideal weight" might be a lot closer than you think. It is now generally agreed that, for many people, a small weight loss, if accomplished through a sensible program, can result in big health benefits—regardless of your present size. Indeed, according to an article by Dr. David J. Goldstein in the *International Journal of Obesity*, many of the health hazards associated with obesity can be alleviated by just a 10 percent weight loss. "For patients who are unable to attain and maintain substantial weight reduction," he writes, "modest weight loss should be recommended."

In fact, perhaps the most significant result of the meeting of obesity and nutrition experts who've put together the most recent set of Dietary Guidelines for Americans is that it was finally conceded that weight *maintenance*, rather than weight *loss*, is a much more realistic goal for most Americans. These 1995 guidelines echo earlier studies that indicated the riskiness of weight gain as we age, but they no longer emphasize the absolute necessity of slimming down to a so-called "desirable" or "ideal" weight. This quiet concession to reality on the part of a government agency is really quite a breakthrough—and a nod to the way many of us, through choice or otherwise, are managing our weight. So if you've been struggling all your life to try to regain your high school figure, it's a struggle you can now abandon without abandoning your health goals.

In the best of all possible worlds, every single one of us would be at our "ideal" weight. We'd all eat right, exercise daily, and no one would smoke cigarettes. We'd all be in glowing health, and we'd be laughing all the way to age 100. However, as we well know, it's not a perfect world, and there's a limit to what each of us can do to improve our lives and our health. Yet the potential for improvement is there—and always has been. Maybe slimming down isn't one of the items on your own to-do list, and that's fine. Just don't use your inability (or lack of desire) to lose weight to keep you from making those other changes that can make you healthier tomorrow than you are today.

PROFILE

Kelly Bliss, M.Ed.

Aston, Pennsylvania
Age: 41
Height: 5'2"
Weight: 200 pounds
Occupation: Personal fitness trainer and psychotherapist

WHEN I WAS IN MY 20S, I was 20 or 30 pounds more than what the height-weight charts said I should weigh, and I put tons of energy into maintaining a low weight. One way I did that was by becoming an instructor in several commercial weight-loss organizations, including Weight Watchers and Diet Workshop. Another way was by developing an eating disorder—I became bulimic. One day, I looked at myself in my bathroom mirror and saw maroon circles, about three inches in diameter, around my eyes. It looked as though I'd been beaten up. It took me a while before I realized that the circles represented millions of tiny broken blood vessels, caused by years of forcing myself to vomit. What I was doing to myself terrified me.

From that day on, I decided to focus on a healthy lifestyle that included nutritious eating, daily exercise—and not worrying about my weight. You see, I had long believed the garbage that society and the medical profession spouted about taking care of yourself, which translated as Being Thin. But once I realized that the only way for me to be thin was to abuse myself and ruin my health, I decided to take care of myself in a way that was right for *me;* being thin was no longer one of my criteria for good health. I was so pleased by the positive changes

PROFILE

I made in my own life and attitude that I decided to go back to school and become both a fitness instructor and psychotherapist working with large people.

These days my eating routine is like this: I eat anything I want at home because I only keep nutritious food in my house—fruit, vegetables, lean meat, fish, chicken, whole grains, sweet potatoes. I usually end up consuming about 1,500 to 1,800 calories a day. I have a real sweet tooth, but I eat sweets only intermittently, such as during a social occasion. That way, they taste much more delicious.

As for my exercise program, I either work out with my clients, teaching an hour-long class that includes aerobics, weight training, and yoga stretching, or else I do personal fitness training where, for two or three sessions a day, I lead people through their low-impact aerobic moves. I may take off a day every couple of weeks or so, but generally, I exercise daily.

I've been following this routine for nearly 10 years now, and since I started, I've gone from about 150 to 200 pounds. That's with daily exercise and no binge eating. I'm one of the millions of people who does "everything right" but whose natural body size isn't what the experts say it will be. I believe it has to do with the set-point theory, which says that the human body seems to have a point—a weight that's healthy for that individual—it will naturally seek when left to its own devices. Nowadays, I live a healthy lifestyle; therefore, I'm at a healthy weight. Remember, too, that I had artificially suppressed my weight for many years. So through a combination of letting my body reclaim its set point and other natural body processes, I got up to 200 pounds. It's a weight I've comfortably maintained, to the penny, for the last four years—through the holidays, when most people gain a few pounds, through a bout with the flu, when most people lose a few pounds, through everything.

PROFILE

When I was in my 20s, the world told me, "If you do such-and-such, you will be thin." But after a decade of doing those things, I realized the world was lying to me. Once I acknowledged that lie, I had two choices: 1) I could go and sit in the back of the bus—meaning, succumb to society's prejudice against fatness and continue to abuse myself in order to maintain a smaller body size; or 2) I could live a healthy life as a full-figured woman. I believe that if I continued to fight my body's natural size, I would eventually have become a statistic—one of those people with cardiovascular disease, gout, high blood pressure, and diabetes. So I decided instead to live a healthy lifestyle and be a naturally large person. Today, I would say I'm a walking commercial for large-size fitness. Most people look at me and assume I'm a size 14 or 16 because of how toned my body is and how well I take care of myself, but I'm actually a size 22.

I believe that if you want to minimize your exposure to society's fat prejudice, you can. How? By developing the confidence that comes from knowing that you're an active, mobile person and that you take care of yourself. Not only will it be physically easier to move your weight through space, but it will be emotionally easier to live in society. After all, if society says, "You're a fat, lazy slob," and you know you worked out an hour today, it's easier to tell society, "You are wrong!" Look, we all know that someone who's 120 pounds and totally sedentary will never be accused of being bad or slovenly, or lazy, the way we large-size people are. That's just the way it is. But that might actually be a blessing, because whatever forces you to look clearly at yourself and your environment and make healthy choices is a good thing. For many people, it's painful and hurtful to be large. But others consider it one of life's greatest lessons on how to take care of themselves.

We all have the right and the responsibility to treat ourselves

PROFILE

well, and by that I mean eating healthfully, engaging in some type of physical activity, and nurturing our self-esteem. If you do those three things the best you can each day, whatever size your body is is the right size for you.

PROFILE

Gordon Elliott

New York, New York
Age: 40
Height: 6'7"
Weight: 255 pounds
Occupation: Talk-show host

I'VE ALWAYS BEEN FIT AND HEALTHY, but at no time in my life, even at my slimmest, was I ever truly happy with my body image. When you're a young guy in your 20s who's 6'7" and over 200 pounds, you want to look like a thin, hip, Ferrari-driving male model, but that just wasn't in my genetic code. I come from a family of robust, very large men—physically, we are the carbon copy of each other. My father is 6'4", and all my uncles are over 6'2"—sturdy, thick-limbed Australian bushmen. My forebears wrestled cattle to the ground for a living!

For a long time, I felt like a relative of Pavarotti's in terms of my size. But now I know I have something more valuable than a thin body: a genetic inheritance of great health. Most of my family has lived into their late 80s, and they've lived well—without cancer or other chronic disease. Most of them were felled by a sudden heart attack. My paternal grandfather, for example, dropped dead after playing three sets of tennis in 120-degree heat in Queensland, Australia. He was close to 80 and would have made it if he hadn't been quite so macho!

I've had ups and downs with my weight. At one point, I was 365 pounds. Then I started working out vigorously and lost more than 100 pounds. I kept that weight for three years, but it was by maintaining an artificial lifestyle—that is, I was constantly lifting weights. The reason I exercise nowadays has

PROFILE

much more to do with how it makes me feel—calm and in control. Today, I weigh 255 pounds. I'm always keeping an eye on my weight because my job is sedentary, and like all the men in my family, I have a tendency to put on weight. So I've got to make sure that physical exercise enters my life on a regular basis. Luckily, I get plenty of exercise thanks to my son, Angus. He is one year old and about 30 pounds and always running around, so it isn't hard. He keeps me very, very active—the days of sleeping in are gone!

As for my diet, it's primarily vegetarian with a lot of fish. I stopped eating red meat seven or eight years ago, and I feel terrific. When I first came to America, I was astounded by the large portions people ate. And everything was so full of sugar and salt—in the bread, in the butter . . . I'm knocked out by the number of additives in foods normally not played with in Australia. My greatest shock after arriving in America was watching daytime television—it was all ads for fast food, followed by ads for laxatives, hemorrhoid creams, and antacids! This country is obsessed with what goes in and out of the body.

I'm careful about the way I eat—I often have grilled salmon and salads. I cut out a lot of the carbohydrates I was eating a year ago, and that's helped bring my weight down. But I can't be a martyr—it creates resentment and leads to overindulging. So once a week, usually Friday or Saturday night, when we're out with friends, I'll have a dinner where I really enjoy myself. That's when I eat whatever I want. But the rest of week, I stick with what I know I should be eating.

I've been married for over two years, and I can honestly say that my weight has had no bearing on our relationship. I've been lucky enough to meet a woman who had a bigger picture of the world than just the way I looked. Sophie herself is blessed with a gorgeous figure and comes from a long line of slender women, but she's not the type to starve or contort her-

PROFILE

self to meet any outside fashion standard. In fact, when I first met her, one of the reasons I knew I'd like her was that she didn't pick at her salad and iced tea—her gusto for food and life was equal to mine. (I'm suspicious of people who pick at their salad—you know there's something else going on.)

And as I've said, my son, Angus, is a big boy. He may be one, but he looks like he's two. He's definitely an Elliott! He'll have to work mending fences in Oklahoma in order to keep slim!

At 40, I'm mindful of having a young son. So I don't smoke or drink much, and I generally keep an eye on my health. I want to be around to enjoy him as long as I possibly can.

Chapter Three

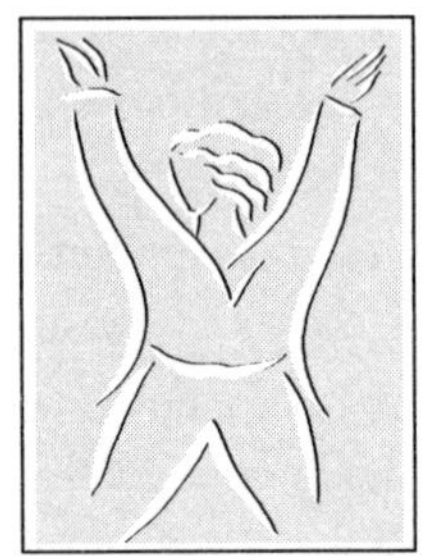

Time for a Change!

If you've stayed with us so far, then you're probably starting to seriously consider making a change for the better in your health. In Chapter Two, we gave you a Personal Health Checklist, designed to help you determine your current health status. Your answers may have led you to the conclusion that everything's okay, that you need do nothing to improve your health. However, as you must realize, health is not merely how you feel *today*, but also how you'll feel—and be—*tomorrow*. In other words, it's also a matter of how much your present lifestyle is helping you preserve or improve your current good health *or* placing you at risk for future health woes.

Therefore, we offer an additional way for you to see whether your health could use some fine-tuning: by consulting the following Risk-Factor Checklist. What's your own level of risk? Ask yourself the following questions.

Risk-Factor Checklist

Lifestyle

1. My diet is probably too high in fat.
Yes____ No____
2. I probably don't eat enough fresh fruits and vegetables and other complex carbohydrates (such as brown rice and whole wheat bread).
Yes____ No____
3. I don't exercise on a regular basis/my lifestyle is basically sedentary.
Yes____ No____
4. I smoke cigarettes/cigars.
Yes____ No____
5. I have difficulty managing my day-to-day stress.
Yes____ No____
6. I use alcohol and/or other drugs to excess.
Yes____ No____
7. I live and/or work in an unhealthy or unsafe environment, e.g., filled with secondhand smoke or high levels of air pollution, etc.
Yes____ No_____
8. I frequently have trouble sleeping.
Yes____ No____

Medical Conditions

1. I have been diagnosed as having an elevated serum-cholesterol level.
Yes____ No____
2. I have been diagnosed as having an elevated level of triglycerides.
Yes____ No____
3. I have been diagnosed as having elevated blood pressure (hypertension).
Yes____ No____

4. I have been diagnosed as having diabetes.
   Yes____ No____
5. I have been diagnosed as having arthritis.
   Yes____ No____
6. I have been diagnosed as having osteoporosis.
   Yes____ No____
7. I have been diagnosed as having chronic lung disease.
   Yes____ No____
8. I have been diagnosed as having heart and/or peripheral vascular disease.
   Yes____ No____

FAMILY HEALTH HISTORY

1. I have a family history of cancer.
   Yes____ No____
2. I have a family history of heart disease.
   Yes____ No____
3. I have a family history of hypertension/stroke.
   Yes____ No____
4. I have a family history of diabetes.
   Yes____ No____
5. I have a family history of arthritis.
   Yes____ No____
6. One or both of my parents are/were obese (which may impact your present weight biologically and/or in your attitude toward food).
   Yes____ No____

Evaluating Your Answers

IF YOU'RE LIKE MOST PEOPLE, you probably checked off at least one Yes answer above—perhaps more than one Yes in each of the three categories. Even if you've decided you cannot or will not do anything further to try to lose weight, you can still take definite measures to improve your health now and lower your risk for ill health later. Make no mistake about it: These are goals well worth setting and reaching, especially because the above-named factors increase your risk of contracting many of the diseases and negative health conditions that appear in the Personal Health Checklist on pages 38-39.

In this book, we'll be focusing on the kinds of habits, customs, and activities listed under the Checklist's Lifestyle heading. These behaviors are the ones that are the most obvious and the most important in terms of your present and future health. Further, they are the ones most directly under your control, the ones you can actively work on to change. You know whether or not you smoke, or how effectively you do (or don't) handle the stressful situations that present themselves to you each day. Once you start tackling the first of the lifestyle-oriented risk factors that you think you can remedy, you'll be astonished by how quickly you'll feel more in control of your life, more energetic, and better about yourself—not to mention all the good you'll be doing in terms of improving your health for life.

Next come the items under the Medical Conditions heading. After lifestyle-oriented risk factors, these are the ones most under your control. For example, if you've undergone a battery of tests suggested by your doctor and have been diagnosed with hypertension, you can then work on ways to lower your blood pressure with methods like better stress management, exercise, and/or a reduction in your sodium intake. If you have high cholesterol, a program of regular exercise and/or a change to a low-fat/low-cholesterol diet may be all it takes to do the trick. We'll be describing ways you can deal with your medical risk factors in Chapters Five, Six, and Seven.

You'll notice, by the way, that we're *not* prescribing a weight-loss diet for easing many of these problems, even though it might help. But if you are reading this book, more than likely you have already tried to do that—on more than one occasion—and it hasn't been the solution. We want to help you shift your focus *away* from weight loss and *toward* those many other things you can do to improve your health. Of course, we all know that healthy lifestyle changes like exercise and an improved diet *may* produce weight loss. But even if they don't, taking these steps will help reduce your level of risk for future ill health—and make you feel better about yourself right now.

As for those items you may have checked under the Family Health History section, it's clear that an inherited tendency toward arthritis, for example, is something you can't undo yourself. Similarly, the fact that a number of close female relatives may have come down with breast cancer puts you, statistically speaking, at higher-than-average risk. These are some facts of life you're going to have to accept. However, knowing your family health history gives you an advantage over others who do not know theirs. Armed with this important information, you can then go back to your answers from the Lifestyle section to see what you can now do to at least reduce your chances of becoming a victim of those family tendencies. For instance, if heart disease runs in your family *and* you currently smoke and lead a sedentary lifestyle, then there are definitely steps you can take—namely, to stop smoking and start exercising—to lower your personal risk for heart disease.

A little knowledge is *not* a dangerous thing. Learning even a bit more about your state of health—and the impact your family history may have upon it—can help you take action to bring those various ill-health risk factors under control.

Enlisting the Help of a Health Professional

AS WE SAID IN THE LAST CHAPTER, you should bring any indication of a serious health problem to the attention of your doctor. You will also need to see a qualified health professional to get many of the kinds of health tests mentioned in the Risk-Factor Checklist, above. Depending on your sex, age, and the date of your last checkup, you may also require such additional tests as a mammogram, Pap smear, and/or rectal exam. (And speaking of your last checkup, if you haven't had one in five years or more, make that appointment today.) Ideally, your doctor should be someone who not only treats illness but also is knowledgeable about evaluating and managing ill-health risks.

While no one considers a doctor's appointment a barrel of laughs, it may be a particularly painful experience for you if you're overweight. This may be especially true if you grew up as an overweight child and have memories of being hounded to lose weight (and possibly ridiculed) by your family doctor. You may have had equally unpleasant experiences as an adult dealing with the medical community. In an attempt to avoid a repetition of those kinds of ordeals, it's possible that you may not have seen a doctor for some time. That's understandable when we realize how remarkably unenlightened many health professionals are about the subject of obesity, how many are quick to blame any and all present and possible future health problems on a patient's overweight, and how many doctors are ready to condemn their overweight patients to a permanent state of ill health if they can't lose weight for one reason or another.

But we know better. If you find that your doctor is simply not on your wavelength when it comes to your weight, find another. Good, sensitive doctors *are* out there, although it may take some time and energy to locate one. Consider calling a number of them and doing a mini-interview with each one over the phone. (In these days of physician oversupply and increasing competition among doctors for patients, the wise doctor will be happy to engage in such a conversation.) Being candid can only help you and your relationship with the physician. Let him or her know that, as a large-size person, you've been unhappy with the treatment you've received in the past from doctors. Ask, "What is *your* attitude toward large-size people?" The answers you get will help steer you to someone who shares your attitudes and wants to help you achieve *your* goals—not his, hers, or society's. The effort will indeed be worth it. You need not put your health at unnecessary risk because you're unhappy with the medical care—or the bedside manner—you've experienced in the past.

Remember, too, that physicians are mere mortals. If you've been raised, as many of us have, to believe that doctors are godlike beings who see all and know all, this may be the perfect time to challenge some medical opinions and procedures you may have secretly disagreed with. For example, you need not automatically get on the scale just because the doctor has asked you to. You can refuse, nicely but firmly, saying something like, "I'd rather not, and since we agreed that you won't be prescribing any weight-loss program for me, I don't believe getting my precise weight is necessary."

There are other ways to assure yourself that the office visit will go smoothly and produce the desired results—elements as basic, for example, as making sure that the blood-pressure cuff placed on your arm is the correct size for you. (A too-small cuff may register a blood-pressure reading that's too high.) These are the kinds of routine doctor's office procedures in which many patients (and doctors!) go on automatic pilot; you may need to be more outspoken about what happens to you.

We'll talk more about self-acceptance and assertiveness later in this book. But for now, even though it may be difficult for you, understand that one of the areas where assertiveness may be most useful in your life is with your doctor. Don't be afraid to question his or her judgments, particularly when you're given a blanket prescription to lose weight "for your health." If all other signs indicate that your overall state of health is fine apart from your weight, you need not attempt to follow this particular piece of advice, especially if a number of past attempts have led to nothing but frustration. Without fear of alienating your doctor, you can clearly indicate that dieting is not something of interest to you at this time (if ever). Steer him or her toward helping you deal with your other risk factors, if you happen to have one or more. Indeed, the more such frank and open discussions are carried on, the more you can help bring your physician's thinking about obesity and obese people into the twenty-first century and beyond.

Should You See a Nutritionist?

You'll notice that questions 1 and 2 under the Lifestyle heading on page 51 deal with matters of nutrition. While you know that we're not advocating weight loss in this book, we *do* recommend that you follow some sort of healthy eating plan to provide your body with the nutrients it needs so that you can feel and function at your best (whether or not you happen to lose weight in doing so). It's also critical to lower a high dietary-fat intake to help head off diseases related to excessive dietary-fat consumption, such as heart disease and certain cancers.

You may already be knowledgeable about what constitutes a healthy diet and may in fact be following such a program. If so, good for you, and keep up the great work! For those of you whose nutritional know-how could use some sprucing up, you'll find in Chapter Five the dietary facts you need to help get your eating on track. As you will see, the food plan we've outlined will assure you of food variety, balance, good taste, and plenty of nutrition.

However, you may decide that you need more—namely, the guidance of a personal nutritionist. As with finding a suitable and simpatico primary health-care professional, it's important that the nutritionist you seek out (should you decide you want one) understands you and your needs—and doesn't automatically hand you a weight-loss diet during your initial visit.

Although you're bound to come across otherwise competent nutritionists who will instantly assume that you're looking for weight-loss advice, there are others who will gladly work with you to help you clean up your poor eating habits without automatically setting weight-loss goals for you. For example, nutritionists who are more concerned with healthy eating than with slim bodies can be found in an organization called AHELP (the Association of Health Enrichment of Large Persons). This group also includes other enlightened physical and mental health-care professionals who are dedicated to the support and acceptance of large people. It might be worth contacting AHELP for a referral (see page 247 for relevant addresses and phone numbers).

Testing, Testing . . .

ONCE YOU FIND A DOCTOR you're comfortable with, you will probably undergo a series of medical tests to help determine your current health status and your health risks, even if you feel perfectly fine. Some doctors, as you may have discovered by now, are somewhat test-happy, routinely administering lab tests whether or not they're truly necessary (or useful). Besides being costly, these tests can occasionally produce false positive results, which will only alarm you needlessly until your correct status has been determined. So it pays for you to know which tests you really need—and at what frequency—and which can be postponed or ignored completely.

Below is a chart you may want to consult before going for your next general physician's or gynecologist's appointment. It lists the *only* lab tests we recommend for adult men and nonpregnant women.

Test	Who should have it?	Optimal frequency
Pap smear (to detect cervical cancer and dysplasia, an abnormality of genital tissues or cells)	All sexually active women over 18	Every 1-3 years
Mammography (to detect breast cancer)	Women over 50 (although many breast cancer experts recommend beginning as early as age 40 and continuing through age 70-79)	Every 1-2 years

Test	Who should have it?	Optimal frequency
Total cholesterol (to detect high blood cholesterol)	Men 35-65 Women 45-65	Every 3-5 years
Fecal occult blood test (to detect colorectal cancer and polyps)	Men and women over 50	Annually
Sigmoidoscopy (to detect colorectal cancer and polyps)	Men and women over 50	Every 3-5 years

Other tests that will probably be given, and should be, include blood pressure, a check of your heart, simple analyses of your blood and urine, and perhaps, depending upon other factors, a test of your blood sugar level. During your meeting with the doctor, it would be beneficial for you to share your findings from the Risk-Factor Checklist on pages 51-52.

What can you expect from a doctor after he or she has administered the necessary tests and discussed the results with you? You should receive concrete information you can use—perhaps a low-fat eating plan to improve your diet, a smoking-cessation or exercise program, a referral to an appropriate community-based program.

With any luck, you will also get some positive encouragement for undertaking the health changes *you* want to make and no negative messages about those you can't or won't make (such as weight loss). What a doctor can't give you, however, is *motivation.* A health-care professional can try a variety of ways and words to help launch you on a healthier lifestyle, but the one who must decide to stop smoking or to lace up those walking shoes three or four times a week is *you.* Truly effective motivation can come only from within. We'll be talking more about how to activate your motivation in the next chapter.

You Know Your Risk Factors— Now What?

YOU'VE GATHERED THE INFORMATION concerning your current risk factors from the checklists above. You've learned the results of your medical tests, ideally accompanied by a few words of guidance from your health professional. Now it's time for you to evaluate all these facts and figures and decide on your next step. The question to ask yourself is, Do I currently have risk factors for ill health? Once you have the answer to that question, your next is, Do I want to do anything about them? Your answer may be no. But if you do decide to work on improving your situation, then you'll want to figure out which problem to tackle first. That is, you'll need to establish your health priorities.

It is a good idea not to try to take on everything at once. For instance, maybe you want to work first on reducing your dietary-fat intake from a current level of about 40 percent of calories from fat to a healthier 30 percent. Great! In Chapter Five, we'll show you how to do that. If, on the other hand, you've decided that the time has come for your cigarettes to walk the plank, that's terrific! In Chapter Seven, you'll find some how-tos to help you kick that habit at long last.

But we strongly urge you to focus on *one* lifestyle change at a time. Why is this so critical? First of all, it's always easier to tackle *anything* in life one step at a time, one problem at a time. You don't want to overwhelm yourself by working on too many challenges simultaneously. Secondly, you'll soon discover that once you are able to deal with one lifestyle problem effectively and make one behavioral change, you're going to learn lessons that you can easily apply to other risk factors. Successfully managing even one health problem means that you are learning many skills: how to mobilize your motivation, become more disciplined, set a schedule, focus on an important, life-enhancing goal, and carry out the specific tasks you need to undertake in order to get there.

In short, by making just one lifestyle improvement, you are learning what it's like to win—possibly after a lifetime of feeling like a loser when it comes to weight loss. Now, you'll finally be able to stop smoking, or learn to create a repertoire of easy, fat-free meals, or start walking three times a week. All of that is *winning*, and it may be a brand-new experience for you—one that can lead to increased self-confidence and self-esteem and to successfully reaching other goals.

Handling Your Own Mental Obstacles to Health Change

OKAY! YOU'RE READY TO CHANGE your health for the better—or *are* you? One look at the present size of your body—and recalling previous unsuccessful attempts to reduce—might lead you to believe that you're incapable of making *any* positive health changes. "If I can't lose weight, how can I expect to quit smoking?" you may be saying. Or, "I've never had success keeping my weight off for any length of time. What makes me think I can stick to an exercise program for more than a week or two?"

While that line of reasoning may be understandable at first glance, here are two thoughts you may not have considered—and indeed, they are among the major premises of this book:

1. **Not all health-behavior changes are the same.**
2. **Some health-behavior-change outcomes can be guaranteed if you follow the recommended procedures, while others, including weight loss, cannot.**

Let's examine these two ideas. First: Not all health-behavior changes are the same. Your past weight-loss frustrations may have convinced you that there's no point in trying to improve other areas of your health, that you will only encounter more failure—and more discouragement and frustration. But what has happened (or, rather, has *not* happened) with your weight is *not* a good indicator of what you can expect if you decide to make other health improvements—quit smoking for good, switch to a healthier diet, or begin a regular exercise program.

Some people find it easier to make a certain kind of lifestyle change than others do. That's because there are so many factors that go into making those changes—personal history and experiences, one's state of mind, biological status, and the needs and demands of one's family, to name just a few.

For example, for a variety of reasons, you may not have been sufficiently motivated in the past to give up cigarettes, but you are now. Fine. Your body's inability to shed pounds has no bearing on your potential success in quitting smoking. Losing weight and quitting smoking are two very different activities involving two distinct sets of behavior patterns. And the good news for those of you who wish to stop smoking is that, overall, the success rate is impressively high. According to the 1993 Surgeon General's report, there's been a 30 to 40 percent reduction in the number of adults who smoke. And Brandeis University's Institute for Health Policy October 1993 report *Substance Abuse: The Nation's Number One Health Problem* reveals that a whopping 48 percent of those over age 20 who have ever smoked in their lifetimes have since quit permanently! Almost half! That's amazingly encouraging for anyone who doubts his ability to succeed at this task. Yet, by comparison, the statistics we have on weight-gain recidivism are staggeringly poor: 90 to 95 percent of us who try to lose weight gain it back.

Weight loss and giving up smoking, weight loss and exercising regularly, weight loss and stress management—these are clearly different challenges, and the truth is that, for many of us, *permanent weight loss is harder and iffier than the others are.* Why? Well, it brings us to our second premise: The outcomes of some health-behavior changes can be guaranteed, while others, including weight loss, cannot. Of all the behavior changes we've named, weight loss is the one where you can do everything "right" and your body may still not respond the way you want it to.

What do we mean? Well, let's take walking as an example. Let's say that your goal is to devote 20 minutes a day, three times a week, to a walking program. Okay, so you've set your goal, and now 20 minutes a day, three times a week, you go out and walk. If you do what you say you'll do, then the outcome of your action is guaranteed. You will have walked, and you will have accomplished your goal. Your achievement is *having done it*, not what the walking can produce (although, chances are, it will, over time, give you quite a few health benefits). The same thing with cigarette smoking. If you either quit "cold turkey" or follow a smoking-cessation program and you do indeed stop smoking forever, that's it! You have become a nonsmoker and will always be one.

But things are very different when it comes to weight loss. No matter whose weight-loss program you follow, no matter how sensible and healthy it may be, no matter how much you slash fat, cut calories, or exercise for hours at a time and follow the program to the letter, there is still no guarantee that you'll lose weight (or keep off any weight you do lose). For reasons we've explained earlier—genetic overweight, very-low-calorie-dieting overweight, a lowered resting metabolic rate, and others—your body may simply not respond to the typical fewer-calories-in/more-calories-burned formula we've been taught will do the trick.

In short, you may do everything "right," and for many reasons, not all of which are understood, you may simply not get the weight-loss outcome you want. Furthermore, a lifetime of trying (and being unable) to achieve that desired outcome can do terrible things to your sense of empowerment and control of your destiny, your self-esteem, and your belief in your ability to succeed in other areas of your life. That state of affairs can be very debilitating and emotionally wrenching for many large-size people.

Remember, however, that the so-called failures we're describing apply *only* to weight loss—and can't even rightly be called failures. So we will say it again: Your past weight-loss attempts are *not* a predictor of the success you can or cannot expect in any other part of your life. The fact is, you have much better results to look forward to in almost every other area! As we pointed out, when you stop smoking, you immediately become an ex-smoker. When you shop for only low-fat or fat-free items in the supermarket (and, of course, eat the items you bring home), you immediately lower your dietary fat. When you start using a treadmill several times a week and keep using it, you have instantly gone from being sedentary to being fairly active and in so doing immediately lower your risk for disease associated with a sedentary lifestyle. See the difference? If only we could be guaranteed those kinds of sure-fire results with our weight by doing all those things we've done for so many years to try to lower it. Regrettably, we can't. It's a sad reality we have to accept—and put aside so we can move on.

Make no mistake, to achieve any permanent health changes requires a keen desire, mobilization of your motivation, and, above all, action. (We've got the recipe for mobilizing your motivation in the next chapter, and all the how-tos you need in subsequent chapters.) Nobody said that quitting smoking or limiting your drinking after a lifetime of three alcoholic beverages a day or giving up those pints of Häagen-Dazs for the sake of your heart is easy. But we urge you: Please stop using your body's inability to cooperate with your desires and genuine efforts to slim down as an excuse to throw in the towel on your total state of health. You have a lot of living to do in the body you currently inhabit. Making that life happier and healthier is definitely within your power.

Handling the Social Obstacles to Health Change

If you are overweight and simply cannot slim down for one reason or another, perhaps the most radical—and the wisest—decision you can make about your life right now is the decision to abandon any further efforts to lose weight and turn your attention to other health improvements. We've already explained why it makes perfect sense to take this bold step, yet it may be a move that others in your life may not be able to comprehend or support. In fact, the biggest obstacle to moving forward with your new health goals may be the very people who love and care about you the most—family, friends, co-workers. As if it weren't bad enough to deal with all of society's messages that Fat is Bad/Unattractive/Unhealthy, now you may be faced with the challenge of dealing with a slim sister or best friend who believes that any other health-improvement efforts you may make are pointless without first losing some weight.

It's never been easy to go against the grain, to make decisions about yourself and your life that are unpopular or nontraditional. It takes self-confidence—self-confidence that may well have slipped away from you during all those frustrating years of being unable to lose weight despite repeated tries. But nobody—not even those people who love you most—know what it is to be *you*, to feel as you do, and have the desires that you have. Now that you've come to the realization that the bottom line is health, not pounds, it should be a bit easier to take the appropriate action, with or without the support of those around you.

In Resources (starting on page 241) you'll find a list of addresses and phone numbers that will help you get in touch with individuals and organizations who share your attitudes and goals. But most important of all is gradually learning to support *yourself*, learning to become your own best cheerleader. Get into the habit of listening to yourself more and respecting your own instincts about what's best for you. The real-life stories of healthy, self-accepting people throughout this book will prove to you that it's possible to take charge of your health with the body you have—regardless of who might tell you otherwise.

Do You Need Psychological Help to Help You Change?

SOMETIMES, WE TRULY WANT TO CHANGE but just can't do it on our own. Realizing that your health could stand some improvement and that you want to make it happen are the most important first steps. But if, for one reason or another, you find that after repeated tries you can't take the next step (with something other than weight loss), then some kind of counseling may be beneficial. Now, we're not saying that psychotherapy is for everyone reading this book. Indeed, if every overweight person who could benefit from therapy got it, the nation's psychotherapists' entire schedule would be taken up with these issues (and there wouldn't be enough therapists to go around anyway!). Furthermore, psychotherapy is beyond the pocketbook of many people.

However, seeking out affordable therapy may be a very good idea if your issues about your weight have brought about real difficulties for you in your day-to-day living. Such situations include:

- feeling down for weeks or months at a time
- having trouble getting out of the house—even to go to work or do other essential activities
- wide mood swings, from down in the dumps to high as a kite
- chronic sleep disorders
- being diagnosed as having an eating disorder
- performing rituals that involve food—for example, obsessively measuring and weighing food right down to the last few grains of rice or cereal (may be a sign of an obsessive-compulsive disorder)
- reading this book but feeling unable to act on any of its suggestions

If you experience one or more of these states of mind and body, it may indicate that counseling would help you move to the next level, both psychologically and physically. You will find references to relevant counseling services in Resources, starting on page 241.

PROFILE

Lynn Meletiche

New York, New York
Age: 52
Height: 5'9"
Weight: Around 350 ("I don't weigh myself")
Occupation: Nurse

I WAS FAT BEGINNING AT AGE 8—I have a long history of battling to attain or maintain the social weight norm. When I was small, my mother dragged me to the doctor, and I was given all kinds of tests. I took thyroid medication for a number of years, and I had injections of unknown substances—my mother doesn't even know what the doctor gave me.

Then, when I was in my teens, I went to a doctor who gave me what was called "rainbow therapy." I'd go once a week, and besides getting an injection of something—diuretics? hormones? who knows?—I'd be sent home with lots of white cardboard boxes filled with pills in a rainbow of colors. There were no names on the pills or the boxes, but I had instructions to take the pink and blue pills when I woke up, and the yellow and lavender pills between meals. Then, when I was in my 20s and out of nursing school, I went on a drug called Eskatrol. I weighed in the low 200s. Eskatrol was a time-release diet capsule, but it was really an amphetamine. I became a terrible person on this medication—I couldn't eat, I couldn't sleep, and I became very nasty and short-tempered. You couldn't even ask me my name without my flying off the handle.

The pattern was always the same: With each successive attempt to get thinner, I would eventually get bigger. I would lose some weight, but then I would gain it back and more,

PROFILE

sometimes double the amount I'd lost.

This pattern continued until I was about 38, when I decided to try a Weight Watchers-type diet. I borrowed the food-plan book from someone and followed the program on my own, without going to the meetings. I was on it for seven months, and I lost 45 pounds. But around that time, my marriage was disintegrating, and I needed to care for my sister, who had been in a bad car accident. I couldn't stop to weigh and measure my food, and over the next six weeks, I gained back 100 pounds!

My weight went over 300 pounds. I may have been eating a bit more than normal—this all took place over Thanksgiving and Christmas—but whatever caused this large and sudden weight gain, I was *not* bingeing. I thought, this weight gain is simply a more dramatic version of what has happened with my weight all my life. And that was the moment I told myself: You can't diet anymore. Lynn, you don't do well with this sort of thing. You've got to stop.

That's when I stopped dieting forever. Since that day, I've just eaten whatever I wanted while trying to eat as healthfully as I can, and over a period of five or six years, my weight finally stabilized. Nowadays, I honor my body's signals, and I eat whatever my body is hungry for; I don't restrict myself according to any diet plan. I'd say I eat between 1,500 and 2,500 calories a day. I may eat at irregular intervals but, again, only when I'm hungry. In fact, I no longer have the desire to eat anything *unless* I'm hungry—when you're dieting all the time, you don't know the difference between feeling hungry and feeling full. But when you give up dieting, you no longer have the food cravings that someone who denies himself may have. In the years since reaching middle age and menopause, I've gained some weight, but it's been very slow and gradual, not like the other times. Generally, I feel very good.

PROFILE

Through this experience, I came to the conclusion on my own that dieting had been destructive for me. Then I heard about NAAFA [National Association to Advance Fat Acceptance], and I joined in 1982. That's when I learned there was a whole body of scientific research that agreed with me, saying that weight-loss dieting simply doesn't work for everyone. I was vindicated! This wasn't just something I had made up to justify myself. It really *was* a phenomenon that affected a lot of people. Not only did that make me feel better, but by becoming involved with others in the same situation, I was able to raise my self-esteem tremendously. Prior to that, I had always felt I wasn't good enough, I wasn't pretty enough, and I certainly wasn't the "right" size. After joining NAAFA, I stopped feeling that way.

Today, I'm vice-president of NAAFA's board of directors. We have 5,000 members nationwide, but that's a drop in the bucket compared with the 58 million fat people in this country. We seem to be preaching to the converted. Why have so few people joined NAAFA? I think it's because most fat people refuse to give up the illusion that someday they'll be thin—they will go to their graves hoping eventually to be a "normal" size—but that can be very damaging to your self-esteem when you see it doesn't happen, year after year. Our members no longer cling to the illusion that we'll be thin someday if we just try harder. We have found greater self-esteem, better health—and a wonderful sense of relief.

PROFILE

Michael Loewy, Ph.D.

San Diego, California
Age: 43
Height: 5'11"
Weight: 320 pounds
Occupation: Psychologist and professor of counseling

I WAS A CHUBBY BABY who became a chubby child. I started dieting before I was 10; my pediatrician gave me amphetamines. Later on, I went to bariatric physicians who put me on very-low-calorie diets. It seemed as if my childhood and adolescence were a series of weight losses and gains—it was always lose 20 or 30 pounds, then put on 25 or 35 pounds. That was pretty much the cycle.

When I was 17 or 18, I went on a no-carbohydrate diet. I lost 50 or 60 pounds and got down to my thinnest adult weight—about 150 or 160 pounds at 5'10". I stayed there until I was 23 or 24, and I started gaining again. Then I started another cycle of dieting—losing and gaining, losing and gaining—until the mid-1980s, when I was in my early 30s. I weighed about 270 at the time, and that's when I went on my last diet, the Beverly Hills Diet. Remember that one? A lot of citrus fruit. I was doing that plus a lot of exercise, and I lost quite a bit of weight, maybe 60 or 70 pounds. I got down to about 200 pounds.

But, as soon as I stopped dieting—what else?—I immediately started gaining the weight back. I was so demoralized and I felt like such a failure—the usual pattern with my eating and dieting. I would diet, lose some weight, gain it back, and feel as if there must be something wrong with me. My life revolved around my diet. I was always thinking about my

PROFILE

diet, my weight, what I should eat, what I shouldn't eat, what I could eat, what I couldn't eat. The whole thing took up so much of my time and energy, and it always left me feeling bad about myself.

This time, though, I came to a decision: to stop dieting. I decided that the struggle was just too painful. I said, That's it! I'm not going to put myself through this anymore. I decided to let myself be what I was. That may sound good, but at the time, it felt as if I was giving up. I had never heard of "size acceptance." I didn't think anyone else felt the way I did. I simply believed that dieting wasn't working for me, so I gave it up, thinking, It's not working, so I'll just forget about it.

It wasn't until later, when I became aware of the size-acceptance movement, that I realized what I had actually done after that last diet was to set myself free from dieting forever. I had been watching "Donahue" one day, and on the show were some NAAFA [National Association to Advance Fat Acceptance] members. I sent away for their literature, and when I read it, I thought, Oh! This is what I need! This is what I've been looking for! It was a whole new concept for me—that one could be fat and healthy as well as fat and happy, and that dieting didn't work for lots of people. I had known it intuitively, but here, for the first time, people were confirming it. Then, in about 1987, I attended my first NAAFA convention in Los Angeles. There I was, surrounded by all these fat people who felt good about themselves, who wore bathing suits and swam in the hotel pool, who felt comfortable. It was the most liberating experience I'd ever had.

Being fat and my struggle with my identity as a fat man has been the most central struggle in my life in terms of coming to grips with who I am as a person. I'm also a gay man, and I had a struggle coming out as gay man and finding a like-minded community there too. That wasn't an easy road ei-

PROFILE

ther. But now, looking at the two issues, I would say that my acceptance of being fat was a more difficult struggle than dealing with my sexual orientation.

Actually, there's a lot of overlap between the two issues—body image and how one sees oneself as a sexual being are closely tied together. The gay community is very body-conscious and very youth-oriented. But even within the gay men's community, there's now a well-organized big men's movement, for large men and their admirers, with clubs and conferences for us in almost every major city in the world. I attend those meetings to help with self-esteem and self-acceptance, and to be around others who appreciate me at my size, not in spite of my size. That is very, very important in terms of dealing with the negative body image many of us have. For me, the process has involved both restructuring negative thoughts about myself—confronting them and actively working to change them—as well as putting myself in environments where I know I will have social support from others on the same path.

There's also the matter of politicizing the issue—seeing fatness not as a personal problem but as a social problem. That has been a very important factor for me in terms of coming out as a gay person and as a fat person. Here, too, the two issues are very similar. As soon as we can stop internalizing the self-hatred and see what we are as the problem of those who try to oppress us—and as soon as we work to change how society thinks about these things instead of trying to change our bodies—the healthier we can become.

I have found acceptance among my friends, but I still have to struggle with certain members of my family. They have a hard time seeing anything but, "Oh, my God, you're fat! You're going to die!" And *that's* from some family members who have weight problems themselves! They're still dieting, so they feel

PROFILE

that at least they're *fighting* their problem, but they think I've just given up, that I'm rationalizing in order to justify being a glutton.

Am I a glutton? No. Sometimes I eat in a healthy way, and sometimes I wish I ate more healthfully. I do not eat compulsively, nor do I overeat in a pathological way, even though for many years I was member of OA [Overeaters Anonymous] because I thought I was a compulsive overeater. At those times when I ate too much, I'd think, I must be a compulsive overeater. But now, looking back, I know that when I ate beyond my satiety, it was in reaction to dieting and a fear of not getting enough food. Since I stopped dieting and reached my current weight about 10 years ago, I've stayed within 10 or 20 pounds of it.

If someone is still having a hard time accepting his or her weight, I would say what they say in 12-step programs—that dieting and your misery will always be there, and you can always go back to them whenever you want, if they make you feel secure. But we all owe it to ourselves to try another way—through self-love. The fact is, some of us were meant to be fat, some were meant to be thin, and some were meant to be medium-size. We can't *all* be thin. We need to change society, not our bodies.

Chapter Four

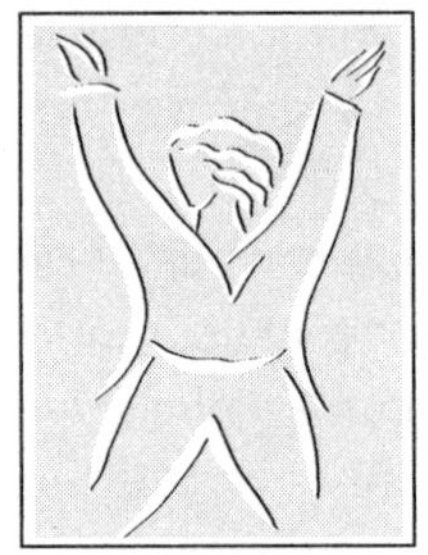

Mobilizing Motivation and Making Permanent Changes

"I'd like about six months' worth of motivation, please . . . " If we could only go to our local mall or tune into the Home Shopping Network and buy a supply of motivation the way we can buy just about anything else. Wouldn't *that* be great? For who among us hasn't said at some time in our lives, "I *know* I could quit smoking/improve my diet/start an exercise program. I've just got to get some motivation."

The fact is, as much as we all toss around the word "motivation," it's actually a poorly understood concept. Motivation isn't some discrete "thing" that comes to us from outside ourselves, something that suddenly, unexpectedly comes over us without warning, like a migraine or an urge for pizza. Motivation is not nearly that unpredictable or whimsical. In most people, motivation is *always* present. That's the good news. The bad news? From time to time, motivation must be *mobilized*, put into action—given a good, swift kick in the pants, if you will. And doing that takes desire and effort on our part.

So it's not a matter of "getting motivated," as so many of us say, but rather *unblocking* our existing motivation, *mobilizing* it. And why is it so critical to do that? Because you can't effect any long-term health changes without it. You need motivation to get going toward your goals and *keep* going long enough to reach and sustain them. Motivation is powerfully energizing; lack of motivation is immobilizing and can be paralyzing.

What Is Motivation?

BEFORE WE GO MUCH FURTHER, we should define exactly what is meant by motivation. Motivation is a *state of mind*, characterized as an emotion, feeling, desire, or idea, *or* a psychological, physiological, or health need mediated by a conscious or unconscious mental process, either of which leads us to take one or more actions. More briefly, it's the process that connects a thought or a feeling to a related action. The root of the word "motivation"—"motive"—actually has two meanings. Originally it meant "moving," which makes sense: motivation gets you moving. In time, however, "motivation" came to take on an additional meaning: the dominant factor in the mental process that causes a person to act.

So what does all this have to do with *your* quitting smoking or signing up for tennis lessons? Two things: 1) talk is cheap; motivation must involve *action* if it is to mean anything, and 2) motivation must originate within you and your own mind and will; nobody else can give it to you.

Weight-Loss Motivation

YOUR PREVIOUS EXPERIENCE with motivation for weight loss may have an impact on your motivation to engage in other health-promoting behaviors now. We *know* you've experienced active weight-loss motivation—that exciting, this-time-I'm-gonna-do-it-nothing-can-stop-me-now sensation. Some of you may have had that feeling many, many times. Chances are, you were able, at least once or twice, to translate that powerful motivation into action: cutting back on your calories or fat intake, increasing your exercise, maybe even keeping a chart of your food intake or exercise—the typical weight-loss routine. And what became of your feelings of motivation, your commitment to your program, after it became clear to you that weight loss was *not*, for whatever reason, happening? Our guess is that your motivation vanished. After all, what could possibly *keep* you motivated if all your hard work wasn't giving you the hoped-for payoff?

So now you may be wondering whether you can ever stir up those old feelings of motivation again when they haven't led to success in the weight-loss arena. The answer is a resounding Yes! As we explained in the previous chapter, body weight is one of those tricky things that doesn't always respond to the tried-and-true methods for taking it off. That's something you understand now. Yet that situation—repeatedly trying to lose weight, without success (and possibly adding *more* pounds than you had before)—may have had a lasting and negative impact on your motivation to change in general. But remember, you *did* get motivated to lose weight. It's just that what you were trying to achieve was not in the cards for you, through no fault of your own. And there are other changes you can make that *can* work for you, such as quitting smoking or starting to exercise—if you can mobilize your motivation once more.

Again, we urge you to put your lack of weight-loss success behind you for the sake of your present and future health. Whatever your weight and weight-loss history, effective motivation to make your health dreams a reality can be yours today.

Motivation and the Process of Change:

The Six Stages of Change and Making Them Work for You

If you've always believed that you were either motivated or unmotivated at any given time—like having an internal on/off switch—then you'll probably be surprised to learn that there are actually various *stages* we go through during the process of mobilizing motivation and making positive change. Psychologists James O. Prochaska, John C. Norcross, and Carlo DiClemente, co-authors of *Changing for Good*, have identified six distinct stages of change: precontemplation, contemplation, preparation, action, maintenance, and termination. Understanding these stages in terms of healthy change can help you monitor your progress and let you see what areas may need some extra effort.

Precontemplation. At this stage, you resist change; you may not even believe you *have* a health problem. If you *are* aware that a health problem exists, you accept it, happily or otherwise. If anyone's doing any complaining about your health, it's probably your spouse, children, or best friend.

Contemplation. Here, you've progressed from the what-me-worry? precontemplation stage to acknowledging there is indeed a problem to remedy. And you'd *like* to remedy it, ideally within the next few months—but how? Your mantra at this stage may be, "I want to stop feeling so stuck." There you are, thinking how great it would be to finally start exercising, how good it would be for your heart, how much it would help tone your muscles—and *then* you start thinking about the way you look in Spandex, how expensive it is to join a gym, how quickly you get winded . . . For every reason you can come up with to make the change, you can produce an equally compelling reason to forget the whole thing.

You *could* go on feeling this kind of ambivalence for years. (If you spend all your time thinking instead of taking action, you're called a chronic contemplator—sort of like the 45-year-old who's been working on his Ph.D. dissertation for the last 20 years.) However, you know the tide has turned when two things happen: 1) you start thinking more about the solution to your health problem than the problem itself, and 2) you start thinking more about your future than your past.

Preparation. Now you're much more committed to making that health change than ever. Sure, there might be little twinges of doubt here and there—I'm *really* going to miss that cigarette with my morning cup of coffee or What's going to happen to my exercise program when I'm on vacation this summer?—but by and large, you're psyched to change your ways, probably as early as this month. Announcing your plan to other people—for example, "Starting next Monday, I'm going on a low-fat eating program"—is a good idea; it will help reinforce your commitment to yourself.

Right now, the importance of making a *specific program* that you will follow can't be overstated. A slow, steady gathering of information and a detailed plan of action for yourself will help you to take control and reach your goals. And keep this thought in mind as you proceed: Gradual change leads to permanent changes. Although some folks who quit cold turkey when they give up smoking or red meat are successful, most people do better with well-thought-out plans that require time to accomplish, according to Prochaska, Norcross, and DiClemente.

Action. This is the stage when, given your high level of motivation to change, Sara Lee cheesecakes and half-empty cigarette packs are apt to be tossed with abandon out of open windows onto unsuspecting passersby. You're cleaning up your act, and in doing so, you've transformed yourself into a whirlwind of activity. You're now exercising regularly, or practicing yoga and deep breathing for stress management, or faithfully keeping that food diary to make sure you're eating all your fresh fruits and vegetables. (*And* you're probably skipping ahead to future chapters in this book to get all the how-tos you need—*that's* how motivated you've become.) Here, too, is the stage where you're not only taking concrete steps to improve your health as needed, but you're probably also starting to change your self-image and your thinking about your future, most likely for the better. A nice bonus: You may be starting to hear some unsolicited words of praise for the healthy direction you're moving in.

Maintenance. Anyone with a dramatic weight-loss history knows that the weight-loss part is a cinch compared with maintaining it. But the maintenance of whatever health habit you're currently working on may well be far easier. The news is very encouraging. Even if you've never been able to maintain your ideal weight for any length of time, you may be much more successful in keeping cigarettes out of your life or sticking to a healthy eating plan or finding a sport you enjoy playing several times a week.

There are two tricky patches to watch out for in the maintenance phase: lapse and relapse. A lapse is a temporary backsliding from which you quickly bounce back to your healthy routine (in exercise terms, the equivalent of taking two to four weeks off). A relapse is a more serious, long-lasting departure from the good health habits you've been engaging in (such as taking up smoking again after being smoke-free for six months).

Lapses are nothing to get too upset about. Look at the bright side: they can be beneficial (by giving your body a rest), and they won't have any permanent deleterious effects as long as your improved health behaviors are fairly ingrained and you return to them promptly. Even relapses can be dealt with successfully. Many people have done it. Simply view that time-out period as a sign that you just weren't as motivated to change as you may have originally thought. Wait awhile, then review the earlier steps we've outlined here. Chances are, you'll get back on track and reach your goal of permanent change.

Termination. This stage should really be called "Hooray!" It's the point you had hoped you'd reach when you first set out to take control of your health. Here's where you "terminate" the struggle to quit smoking or keep working out. Indeed, by now you feel so good and good about yourself—and the new habits are so much a part of your life—that you wouldn't dream of ever picking up a cigarette or missing more than a week or two of exercise. No one's talking about perfectionism here, simply the feeling of mastery and control that says that you have won your battle against sedentary living or poor nutrition or smoking or unmanaged stress.

You've truly changed for the healthier—and the changes feel very, very good.

Internal vs. External Motivation and the Power of Belief

FROM OUR DISCUSSION OF MOTIVATION so far, it should be fairly clear that the most powerful drive leading you to make any change for the better comes from one person: *you.* However, in the past, you may not have had this compelling *internal motivation.* During previous attempts to lose weight, for example, you may have found that your primary goal was to slim down for the sake of someone else in your life—a spouse, a concerned friend or sibling, a child. Or possibly there was an important event you had to look especially good for—a class reunion, perhaps, or a vacation where you wanted to fit comfortably in revealing clothes.

It may have worked—but for how *long*? If you're reading this book, chances are the weight loss wasn't permanent, and little wonder. When any action is taken to please someone other than yourself or to get ready for a particular event on the horizon, that's called *external motivation.* Unfortunately, studies have found time and again that only when you're *internally* motivated to change because *you* have decided it's important will you be likely to reach the goals you've set for yourself.

Are you wondering whether the motivation you have now to make some of those health changes is based on internal or external factors? Look at the statements below. Which ones sound most like you?

1. "Rob threatened to divorce me if I don't stop smoking in bed."

2. "My doctor told me I need to get some exercise. Maybe she's right."

3. "My stress level is ridiculous, and it's been this way for months. I've got to deal with it—now."

4. "I'm always so tired, and I get easily winded too. I'm only 33 years old, but I feel closer to 60. I don't want to live this way for the rest of my life."

It's not too tough to figure out that Speaker #1 and Speaker #2 are driven by external motivation—the wishes or suggestions of others—while Speaker #3 and Speaker #4 are internally motivated. They might all *begin* to change their health behaviors at the same time and with the same urgency in their voices and actions—but check back with them in six months. It's highly likely #1 and #2 will still be smoking and sedentary, while #3 and #4 may be well on their way to healthier, more satisfying lives.

One more thing about your ability to effect change. In the midst of all this motivation talk, please remember that any long-lasting change must also be accompanied by another key ingredient: *belief,* your unswerving faith that you can indeed accomplish this positive change. You must be utterly convinced—despite past frustrations with weight loss, despite what other people say is possible or impossible, despite statistics indicating that the odds may be against you—that you're going to do it, that you're going to be able to take control and succeed where others may have failed. That positive attitude will see you through to your goal and beyond.

The Natural History of Health and Healthy Change

IN THE FIELD OF MEDICINE, we say that there's a natural history of disease. By this we mean that any and all diseases follow a path that explains a patient's present physical condition. Let's take a patient with heart disease. It probably started some time ago with the laying down of plaque on his coronary arteries (a hardening and thickening on the walls of the tubes that carry blood to the heart's own muscle), a process possibly brought on by a high-fat diet and a sedentary lifestyle. His disease may then have progressed to the point where a small blockage developed in one of the arteries. That would have caused a part of the heart to weaken and die. Over time, this patient will probably experience a slow, gradual decline in his heart function. If nothing is done to reverse the trend, he may well die prematurely of heart disease. Just as we've done here with our heart-disease patient, we could trace a disease history for a patient with cancer, diabetes, stroke—in fact, for just about any disease you can name.

Similarly speaking, there is a natural history of *health*—that is, being in a state of health also means a path has been followed. When a person is generally healthy, that path may have included such stages as understanding, determining, and then controlling risk factors; maintaining a positive mental attitude; and having regular health-status screenings, leading to the early detection and successful treatment of disease.

Part of the nature of health is that you can never "finish the job" or reach a state of perfect health; you can only strive for it. That process of striving for better health, in fact, is itself healthy, because your state of mind is positively involved in making you healthier and because you're doing things that improve your body little by little.

But that's one of the interesting aspects of becoming and staying healthy: while it's a never-ending process, you can and should set and plan to reach intermediate goals along the way as you travel on your journey. For example, if you're currently a fairly sedentary person and you wish to become a regular exerciser, then exercising a certain amount each week means you've achieved a *weekly* fitness goal, which is building toward your overall goal to become a regular exerciser. If you hope to reduce your usual fat intake from 40 percent to 25 percent, then cutting down your red-meat meals from five a week to four and then three and then two means you're reaching a *weekly* fat-lowering goal while working toward your overall goal of a 25-percent-fat diet. Observing yourself reaching those intermediate, finite goals along the way gives a wonderful sense of satisfaction and helps keep motivation high.

Are You Ready to Change for Good?

YOU'VE DETERMINED YOUR HEALTH STATUS by answering the questions in Chapter One. You've checked out your risk factors in Chapter Two. You may have seen a doctor for a checkup and some blood tests, and you have a pretty good idea about what areas of your health need work. Earlier, you may recall, we recommended that you take things one step at a time, that you resist any urge you may feel to overhaul your health all at once. At the same time, you might still be experiencing some twinges of doubt about whether you're ready to take those baby steps that lead to permanent health changes. Maybe you're ready—but maybe you're not. Answering these questions should help:

1. Would you like to make a change in your health?
   Yes____ No____
2. Would you like to make a change in your health now?
   Yes____ No____
3. If you answered Yes to question 2, would you like to make a big health change now?
   Yes____ No____

4. If you answered Yes to question 2, would you prefer to make a little health change now?

Yes____ No____

5. If you answered No to question 2, do you think you might be more motivated to get started in a few months?

Yes____ No____

6. Even if you answered Yes to questions 1 or 2, do you believe that you're capable of making some sort of health change now?

Yes____ No____

7. If you answered Yes to question 5, do you believe that you're capable of making a big health change now?

Yes____ No____

8. If you answered Yes to question 5, do you believe you are only able to make a little health change now?

Yes____ No____

9. Do you believe you would be satisfied if you could achieve just one small improvement in your health now?

Yes____ No____

10. Have you ever made a positive change in your life that you can now use as a model to help you make the health change(s) you want to make?

Yes____ No____

11. Do you now have the encouragement and support of others for your desire to make a health change?

Yes____ No____

12. Do you believe you can make the necessary sacrifices (of time, of giving up something you enjoy like smoking, etc.) in order to improve your health?

Yes____ No____

These questions have no right or wrong answers. But the answers you come up with will give you a pretty good idea whether you're psychologically and emotionally prepared now to set your goals, make a real commitment to yourself, take control, and start down the path to reach your personal finish line. It isn't even necessary for you to analyze all your reasons for working on your health;

for now, simply acknowledge and respect your feelings. Are you *feeling* ready?

Again, we realize that you may be facing a mental or emotional roadblock resulting from your past frustrations with weight loss. We want to help you remove that roadblock by reminding you, once again, that you don't have to lose weight to be healthy. And we also want to remind you that if, in your personal natural history of health, you're not ready to start today, you may be ready in three, six, or twelve months.

Goal-Setting: Why It's Critical to Health Change

IT'S IMPOSSIBLE TO OVEREMPHASIZE the importance of setting goals for yourself. What are goals? They are the answers to such questions as What is it that I want to do? and Why do I want to do it? The goals you set for yourself should be realistic ones for you, but they won't mean much unless they require some significant effort on your part to reach them. For many people, goal-setting—knowing what *you* want to accomplish and *why* you want to accomplish it—is the single most crucial element in effecting change. Why? Because that knowledge empowers you, puts you in control, and makes it possible for you to move forward—you *know* where you are going. Goal-setting is the best way to mobilize your motivation. Spend some serious time thinking about the answers to the questions we have posed above. You will find that time well spent.

Again, we urge you to start small. Zero in on one simple behavior change, or even *part* of a behavior change, you can make. There will be more specific how-tos in upcoming chapters, but for now, consider these suggestions:

• **If starting an exercise program seems too overwhelming right now . . .** make it a goal to walk once a week, or get off the bus one stop before your normal one and walk the rest of the way, or park your car as far away as you can from your office building and still be in the company lot.

• **If giving up cigarettes seems too overwhelming right now . . .** make it a goal to cut back by one smoke in every five.

• **If eating a healthier diet seems too overwhelming right now . . .** go to the supermarket this week and substitute two new low-fat or fat-free products for high-fat products you usually buy.

• **If working on stress management seems too overwhelming right now . . .** make a goal to do a week's worth of simple deep breathing for just three minutes a day while seated in a comfortable chair.

• **If improving your total personal-safety environment seems too overwhelming right now . . .** make it your goal to fasten your seat belt every time you drive your car during the next week.

Many people find it helpful to write down their goals in some kind of notebook where they can easily be found, reread, and updated as needed. Jotting down your goals will help you determine what is it you want to do ("Lower the fat in my diet," for instance) and why you want to do it ("To feel better and less sluggish, to cut my risk of heart disease and lower my cholesterol").

Determine if your goal seems reasonable for you to do now. For example, if there is a lot of upheaval in your current daily routine — your sister and her young kids have temporarily moved into your house, say—then this might not be an ideal time for you to do heavy-duty fat-gram calculations for every meal. But maybe your fat-cutting goal for *now* might be simply to buy a few more low-fat products or to cook without added fat or oil for the next few meals or to avoid fast-food restaurants for a week. Writing down your goals will also help you establish what supplies or information you'll need to reach them. We call these "facilitating factors." Do you intend to go swimming twice a week, but you don't know what the new hours of your community pool are? That information is a *facilitating factor*, and you will need to find it out. If part of your stress-lowering program is taking a yoga class, will you need special clothing? It, too, is a facilitating factor you will have to provide.

For each goal, you might want to describe one or more objectives that are specific, measurable actions you can take to achieve the goal. Then, set a time frame during which you can reasonably complete each action. For example, you could set a goal of "becoming a regular exerciser." An objective to accomplish in helping you reach that goal is "walking three times a week, for 20 minutes at a time, by one month from now." If at that time you decide you want to do more, set another objective, always keeping in mind these ideas: "Explore your limits; recognize your limitations" and "Gradual change leads to permanent changes." From there, who knows how much you can achieve?

Most people can do *something* to improve their lives and their health. For starters, choose something you *think* you can succeed at. Success is so much of a better motivator than failure, even if it is a small success at the beginning. Starting small is a very good way to end up with big, satisfying results.

And what if you just can't do anything now? That's fine too. As we said earlier in this chapter, you're simply not there yet in your natural history of health. You're not ready yet. Don't get discouraged. Pick up this book again in three months. Who knows? Your life—and your outlook—may have changed, and you may be raring to go.

Making a Contract for Change

FEW THINGS ARE AS HELPFUL to the change process as writing things down. Earlier, we suggested that you jot down your health-change goals. Here, we're recommending that you draw up a "contract" with yourself. In doing so, you will be taking yet another step in the positive-change process. It's not a legal document, of course, but it may prove to be extraordinarily effective in making your promises to yourself and the goals you set for yourself doable and, in time, a reality.

If you want to make the contract *only* with yourself, that's fine. Alternatively, you might want to include others in your contract, getting them to make a corresponding commitment to help you make the changes you want to make. Do whatever you think will work best for *you.* On the facing page is a sample contract for someone who wants to quit smoking. It involves not only the person who wants to make the change but also friends, family members, and the smoker's health-care provider.

As you can see, this contract is general enough so that it can be adapted to any of your health-behavior goals. After it's been filled out and signed by all the appropriate parties, you might decide to put it away somewhere and not look at it again until the date you set for completion of the project. Or, you might find it helpful to look at it weekly or monthly, to remind yourself of your goal(s) and of the support being offered to you in your efforts. You might even want to write a reward into your contract that you will give yourself upon the successful attainment of your goal or interim goals. Depending on how high your degree of motivation is right now, this little piece of paper has the power to literally change your life. Try it; what do you have to lose?

Dealing with Flagging Motivation

NO MATTER HOW HIGH YOUR MOTIVATION to change is at the beginning, no matter how well-thought-out your program, there will likely be a time when your motivation starts to sag. It may come suddenly, as a surprise to you (What happened? you'll think. I was so fired-up last month!). Or it may be the result of a slow, creeping feeling that comes over you, the sense that it's all too much trouble for too little (or too slow) a pay-off. This is a common experience, especially if you're one of those people who went on crash diets in the past.

If you started out with a lot of weight to lose, a crash diet may have enabled you to drop double-digit poundage in a matter of *days.* Talk about instant gratification! But what happened? Did the weight

Sample Contract for Quitting Smoking

Name *Jane Harrison* Date *3/30/96*

My health goal is to *give up all smoking*

by *Sept. 1* 199 *6*

Steps I will take to achieve my goal:

By April 15, I will reduce my 2-pack-a-day smoking to 1 and I will go on nicotine patches and stop all smoking.

Steps my family/friends have agreed to take to help me:

They won't smoke in my presence for the next 6 months and they will give me every encouragement.

Steps my doctor (other caregiver) has agreed to take to help me:

(1.) Give me all the directions and encouragement I need. (2.) Answer my questions (3.) Provide prescriptions needed (4.) Be patient if I backslide (5.) Put gentle, consistent pressure on me

If I don't achieve my goal, in addition to the negative health consequences, I recognize that *it will be up to me to admit the difficulties I'm having and to make every effort to try again.*

Signed: *Jane Harrison* Date *3/30/96*

Paul Harrison Date *3/30/96*

(family member/friend)

[signature] Date *4-2-96*

(doctor/caregiver)

stay off? Probably not. And it's possible you went on to some other, equally ill-conceived diet. So you're very experienced with diets that don't work, and at some point, you might doubt that anything this book encourages you to do will work, either.

However, nobody is suggesting that you can expect to go from couch potato to athlete in a week or from two-pack-a-day smoker to nonsmoker overnight. We are endorsing slow, steady *lifestyle* changes, the kind that produce slow, steady, *lifelong* improvements. With that comes the sometimes painful realization that most of the changes will take a while to see and feel. That means keeping your motivation mobilized, even when it might start to flag—a perfectly natural stage in the process. And *that* means a commitment on your part to hang in there on those freezing-cold mornings when you don't want to get out of bed, much less exercise for 30 minutes. It means not getting careless about your newfound healthy-eating program when there's a family crisis. And it means being true to the promise you made yourself to stop smoking for the sake of your health, even though the gang is going out for Happy Hour and the air is thick with cigarette smoke.

The fact is, sooner or later Real Life is going to intrude on your health plans. The question is, How are you going to handle it? By being prepared for that inevitable occurrence. One way to do so, perhaps, is to decide ahead of time that, if absolutely necessary, you'll give yourself an occasional break from your program, but that you'll quickly return to it because you know that reaching your health-behavior goals is vitally important to you.

That's the key: *making the decision and taking control of your actions.* It means you won't be tossing your goals aside because they're too hard or because what everyone else is doing looks like more fun; nor will you get down on yourself and give up because you occasionally take a "time out" from your program. That's okay as long as it's just a time out—and not an end-of-game. It isn't always easy to sustain your health-promoting activities. But once you mobilize your motivation again, you know that the physical and mental rewards for doing so will be well worth the effort.

So, okay, you skipped your morning run today or you didn't

floss your teeth—life goes on, and you've done minimal damage. Maybe your desire to slough off a bit is a sign that you're trying to do too much too soon, or that you need a break. Knowing when to give yourself a rest is as important as creating the most wonderful exercise program or low-fat eating plan. As long as you're in control of the situation, fine. Control—being in control and staying in control—is central to your success; it's at the heart of succeeding in all of these behavior changes you're trying to make for a happier, longer life. No one's running this particular show but *you.* You decide what you'll do and how much. Knowing when to temporarily stop your program—as well as starting and sustaining it again—will ensure your long-term success.

Should You Join a Motivation-Boosting Group?

DO YOU NEED TO JOIN a smoking-cessation group to kick the habit for good, or can you gradually wean yourself off cigarettes? Will power-walking with a group of friends get you going in the morning, or would you prefer to spend your exercise time as a private time for communing with nature or just getting more in touch with yourself?

As with the questions we asked above concerning your readiness to change, there's no right or wrong answer here, either. It has been shown that people are often more successful at making lasting changes when they get the support and encouragement of like-minded people. However, you may be the type of person who prefers to exercise at your own pace (and listening to the kind of music *you*, not a fitness instructor, choose). An organization such as NAAFA (National Association to Advance Fat Acceptance) or Abundia, based in Aurora, Illinois (see Resources, page 247) may be worth joining if you're still having trouble accepting the idea of getting fit while staying fat and could use the support of other large-size women and men. On the other hand, you may already be at the stage where you accept your body size and are ready to make other improvements.

The bottom line? Mobilize your motivation and set your goals—these processes are interrelated and often go on together. What is it that *you* want to do and why do you want it? Often, answering these questions, spending some real time thinking about your answers, and accepting them for yourself is all you need to do to unblock your motivation—and then get going.

PROFILE

Willard Scott

Delaplane, Virginia
Age: 62
Height: 6'3"
Weight: 252 pounds
Occupation: "Today" show personality

GROWING UP, I was pretty much at a normal weight until I hit 18 and went to college. I had always liked to eat, and I guess my metabolism began to change. Within six months of starting college, I went from 150 pounds to 165 pounds. That was the first wave of weight gain.

Since then, I've excelled in one thing: being consistent at gaining weight! In time, I reached 312 pounds, but I never worried about it because I've been so active and healthy, thank God. I've been blessed—I don't have diabetes, high blood pressure, high cholesterol, or any other problems associated with overweight. I've never had any real reason to lose weight, except maybe my pride. Oh, and I guess I might've wanted to look good because I appear on television every morning. But honestly, my weight never bothered me. Sure, every now and then someone—a doctor or a fan—would say (in a nice way), "Willard, you're so nice. You should lose weight for your own good." But I never really felt like it.

Then, a few years ago, someone from SlimFast contacted me and asked if I would do a commercial. I said, "No, I'm just not motivated to lose the weight." But then he called again, and finally I went on SlimFast and did the commercials. I was on a modified version of the program—I added some extra food here and there. It's a good supplement, and it did help

PROFILE

me lose weight. But what really triggered my desire to lose weight was that four years ago, my grandson was born, and I started thinking about my mortality. It wasn't the fact that I was on television or getting up to 312 pounds or having a hard time finding clothes and having to buy them at the Gorilla Shop. The real catalyst was the birth of little John Willard.

I waited till my late 50s to do something about my weight, but the fact is, I've *always* been very happy with myself, even when I was bigger. Without sounding like an egomaniac, I would say I have no major hang-ups. I love people, and I want people to love me. If I have any obsession other than food, it's the desire to be loved. The key to a healthy body is a healthy mind and being surrounded by love. That makes all the difference in how you feel about yourself, whatever your weight. Liking yourself has to do with the people around you, who love you for *you.* And if you are loved and you love others, it will create a sense of well-being that will let you feel okay with the way you are.

If you're basically healthy, as I am, I don't think you should be obsessed with getting on the scale every day—I only weigh myself once every three months or so. And if you're on a healthy food plan, don't worry if you go off it sometimes. I think it's okay once in a while to eat two chocolate sundaes if you really want to. Then watch yourself the rest of the time. You *don't* have to torture yourself or give up what you enjoy. For example, every week, I still have a steak and a baked potato—but now, instead of putting sour cream on the potato, I use salsa. There are so many things you can substitute and still give yourself the foods you love most. One of my problems is that I'm on the road so much, where the food may be different from what I'd normally eat. But when I'm at home, I have total control; I have really cut back on my fat. Plus, my wife Mary is a dedicated weight watcher—she's very conscious of

PROFILE

her weight and her health. She's basically on the Pritikin program, and eating my meals with her generally means I'm eating healthy.

I also try to be active. We live on a farm, and when the weather's good, I'm in the yard raking, gardening, hoeing . . . In the summertime, I usually lose 8 to 10 pounds without even trying. I also like to ride a bike—a *real* bike, not an exercise bike—and swim. Sleep is so important too. Because I have to get up at 4:00 A.M. for the "Today" show, I get my sleep in two sessions, but it adds up to around six and a half or seven hours a day.

I think we've come full circle in our attitude about weight. We know we don't have to be Twiggy. We are all so different, and some people just weren't made to be thin. What you want to be is healthy and make your body totally responsive so that you can do what you want to do. Far more important than the way you look is the way you feel.

Chapter Five

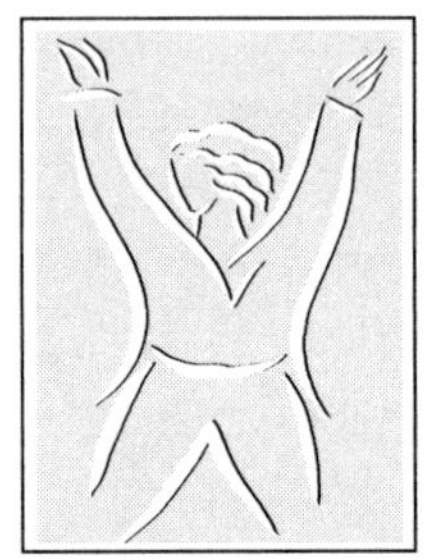

The Big Picture Plan *for* Health: Eating

If you're like most large-size people, you probably consider D-I-E-T a four-letter word—and for good reason. Most of the diets we read or hear about—in women's magazines, in diet books, on talk shows—are full of hope and promise of guaranteed weight loss in a matter of days or weeks. But as you well know, the vast majority of them do little to shrink our size permanently (although they often manage to enlarge the wallets of the diet creators). Chances are, if you're reading this book, you've been on and off weight-loss diets much of your life, to little avail. Even if you consistently chose to follow sensible diets and did everything "right," weight loss may just not have happened for you, possibly leading to anger, depression, and frustration.

No wonder so many large-size women and men throw in the towel, stop weighing themselves, and vow to eat whatever and whenever they like.

You know by now that this is not a weight-loss diet book; your shelves are bulging with enough of those by now (that is, if you haven't burned them all). But we would certainly be remiss if we talked about getting healthy without a discussion of healthy eating. Again, we're *not* talking about a diet with the aim of getting you to shed pounds. We're talking about delicious, easy-to-fix, healthful foods and balanced, nutritious meals that can become the basis of a lifetime eating plan.

Why is smart eating such a smart idea? There are two reasons. First, in order to live comfortably with your present weight, it's good to eat sensibly. You may feel fine about your size right now, but at the same time, you'd probably be wise to not let it get out of hand. Whatever your weight, it's best to maintain it rather than increase it. D-I-E-T may be a four-letter word to you, but the phrase "weight control" should definitely not be dismissed. You may feel fine today, but you may not feel so terrific with another 50 or 75 pounds on your body.

Second, regardless of your weight, unhealthy eating habits, such as consuming a high-fat diet, can shorten or reduce the quality of your life by increasing your risk for health problems like high cholesterol, heart disease, or cancer. (By the way, we *do* use the D-word throughout this chapter, but when we do, we're referring to a *way of eating*, not another quick-fix weight-loss program.)

So if you think that choosing simply to maintain your weight means eating whatever happens to be in front of you (or in the nearest vending machine), think again. Your weight is one thing; your health is another. And good nutrition is one of the primary ways that you can control the state of your health for the rest of your life.

Eating for Health (Instead of for Weight Loss)

CHANGING ANY UNWANTED BEHAVIOR involves some thinking, planning, and mobilizing of your motivation, as we discussed at length in the previous chapter. Yet you're about to discover that eating right for the sake of your health—*not* with the express aim of losing weight—is going to (you'll pardon the expression) take a big weight off you (and your mind).

There's something wonderfully liberating about knowing you're improving your nutrition without having to worry about how many pounds you're going to drop this week. You will quickly see that the mental discipline required to shift, say, from a high-fat to a low-fat diet is far less than what is necessary to try to lose X number of pounds. That's because the emphasis is now on your day-to-day behavior, which you *can* control, rather than on how much and how fast you lose weight, which you cannot.

Put another way, the outcome isn't measured by your *weight* but rather what's on your *plate*. What you serve for tonight's dinner, how much oil you use in your cooking, what you shop for in the supermarket, what entree you select from the restaurant menu—all of these actions (and more) will soon translate to a healthier you, regardless of what does or doesn't happen on the bathroom scale. Even if you used to feel helpless and hopeless in the presence of food—believing that food was somehow the enemy—you're going to find out very soon that you can actually be in control of food and make it a truly pleasant and positive part of your life.

The Big Picture Plan for Healthy Eating

EVERY FOOD PROGRAM HAS A NAME, and we're calling ours the Big Picture Plan for Healthy Eating. Why? It's our way of encouraging you to view good nutrition as part of the big picture of health, which also includes regular activity, stress management, eliminating known health risks such as smoking and drinking to excess, and improving personal safety—in short, all the factors that contribute toward improving your state of health. Food is a critical element here—don't get us wrong about that—and yet it's only one slice of the whole low-fat pie.

We know you're going to enjoy this "food plan" because it's one that you structure *for yourself,* not one that's structured for you. And there's no calorie counting, no fat-gram toting, no hand-held calculators. The fact is, most of us can't keep up those routines for long, and anyway, this is intended to be a *lifestyle* change, not a quickie weekend diet that promises to get you into a size-smaller dress by Monday. Mercifully, those days are over. Now, and from now on, you're into eating smart, and you're calling the shots about how you're going to do it.

Your goal—with simple, manageable, intermediate goals along the way—is to achieve a permanent change in the way you approach food, buy food, prepare food, and, of course, eat food. Rules and restrictions will be kept to a minimum. You're going to start making *conscious choices* about what will be on your personal menu. The key is *awareness*—really paying attention to your eating in a way you may not have done up till now—but not obsession. By taking control of your food-related actions—what foods you choose to eat and how much you choose to eat—you can change your daily eating patterns for the healthier. By adjusting your personal menu—from high-fat to lower-fat foods—you'll automatically slash your overall dietary-fat intake. And by keeping an eye on the amounts of food you consume each day, you'll keep your weight steady. By doing these things, you'll be pleasantly surprised by the quantities and range of food you can still enjoy when you focus on minimizing the presence of one little devil in your diet: fat.

Why Go Low-Fat?

IT'S SAFE TO SAY THAT HIGH-FAT DIETS account for most of the food-generated health woes in the world, everything from heart attacks to colon cancer. And since our current focus is on improving your health and lowering your risk of disease through the food you eat, cutting fat is the best way to do it. But, as we've said before, you're not going to drive yourself into a frenzy worrying whether a chicken breast has four or six grams of fat in it. Instead, by shifting the foods in your diet repertoire from generally high-fat items to low- or no-fat ones, you will be able to eat well, feel satisfied, and improve the way you look and feel.

Slowly and gradually—because that's the most effective way to make changes like these—healthy, delicious, low-fat foods will assume permanent places on the menu of your mind. And the best way to imprint this new menu permanently on your consciousness is to create it *yourself*, over time, choosing the low-fat foods you like best. After a while, low-fat eating will be as natural and automatic for you as high-fat eating is for so many other folks.

From the moment you first heard the phrase "low fat," it was probably linked with the phrase "weight loss." And while it's true that low-fat eating does, for some of us, lead to weight loss, the potential benefits of cutting fat in your diet go far beyond what may or may not show up on your scale:

• **Reducing dietary fat, particularly the saturated fats found in animal products like red meat and butter, lowers your blood cholesterol level.** If your cholesterol level is above 200 (milligrams per deciliter), that can lead to atherosclerosis (formerly known as hardening of the arteries, since the artery walls become coated with fatty substances). This, in turn, makes it more difficult for blood to be transported from your heart and lungs to your muscles, nerves, bones, and other body tissues and organs, including your heart. You know what's next: cardiovascular disease and possibly a heart attack.

• **High-fat diets have been associated with increased risk of cancers of the colon and prostate.** While there currently isn't the kind of evidence to indict dietary fat in the promotion of these cancers the way there is with heart disease, experts in the field do agree that limiting fat intake would almost automatically lead to an increase in consumption of healthier foods, including ones known to fight cancer, such as citrus fruits, broccoli, and potatoes (containing vitamin C); leafy green vegetables (containing vitamin E); carrots and sweet potatoes (containing beta-carotene); and fiber-rich whole grains and cabbage.

There are also studies that seem to indicate a link between high-fat diets and an increased incidence of breast cancer, skin cancer, and even lung cancer—another good reason to lower your fat intake. (Even if the proof is so far inconclusive, isn't it better to err on the side of caution and cut that fat?)

• **Reducing fat may reduce your chances of developing diabetes.** You may already know that diabetes is the number-one disease associated with obesity. And while you may or may not be able to do anything about your weight, you *can* help yourself avoid developing diabetes by limiting the amount of saturated fat you eat. One study done in Finland showed that when subjects ate a lot of animal (saturated) fat, it prevented the metabolism of glucose in their body—and impaired glucose tolerance frequently paves the way for Type II (non-insulin-dependent) diabetes.

For those of you who already have diabetes and are overweight, don't despair. According to the National Institute of Diabetes and Digestive and Kidney Diseases, if you can lose *some* weight, you can get better control of your disease. But it isn't necessary to lose a great deal of weight or to slim down to any so-called "ideal weight" to do it. It has been found that losing as little as 5 to 10 percent of your current body weight can be effective enough to make diabetes disappear. So if you *are* motivated to shed some pounds, cutting fat from your diet may be the simplest way to do it.

• **A high-fat diet may impair the functioning of your immune system, some experts believe.** Research shows that auto-immune diseases like rheumatoid arthritis, thyroid disease, lupus, even allergies are related to high-fat diets—another good reason to minimize your dietary fat.

• **Carbohydrates and proteins each contain four calories per gram versus the nine calories per gram you'll find in fats.** As a result, you can eat more than twice as many carbohydrates and protein foods for the same number of calories, which means you'll feel more satisfied.

• **Eating low-fat just makes you feel better.** Very often, people who eat too much fat—a big chocolate bar, say, or a hunk of cheese—wake up the next day feeling engorged and uncomfortable. You're likely to feel much better—less sleepy, sluggish, and heavy—

if you stick to less fat, more carbohydrates, and a moderate amount of protein. Once you see how good you feel on such a diet, you're likely to keep it up.

Dietary Fats: The Good, the Bad, and the Awful

WHILE YOU HEAR US EXTOLLING the importance of eating a low-fat diet, don't get the impression that *no* fat is best of all. Fat is one of the three macronutrients, along with carbohydrate and protein. All the foods you eat contain at least one of these three essential nutrients, and sometimes two or all three. Fat, while needed by the body in far smaller amounts for good health than the other two macronutrients, is nevertheless critical to help keep you at your healthiest. For example, one type of fat, called polyunsaturated fat, provides the essential fatty acids necessary to help the body manufacture hormones, promote cell growth, and, many experts believe, prevent heart disease. Other reasons you need some fat in your diet are:

- to aid in the absorption of fat-soluble vitamins, including vitamins A, D, E, and K, and carrying them to the body where needed
- to provide energy
- to convert beta-carotene to vitamin A
- to help maintain healthy skin and hair
- to help maintain a healthy nervous system
- to slow down the digestion and emptying of food from the stomach, thereby producing a long-lasting sensation of fullness (which we want in moderation)
- to cushion and protect the body's vital organs

So you see why fat is a critical nutrient. However, while all fats and oils are about the same in terms of the energy they provide (14 grams of fat and about 120 calories per tablespoon), they differ in their composition. Some are definitely better for you than others.

If you're confused about the differences, the descriptions below should help:

• **Saturated fat.** This type of fat is found in animal products like red meat, whole milk, whole-milk cheeses, butter, and lard. It is usually in solid form at room temperature, although such liquid fats as palm oil and coconut oil are high in saturated fat too. Manufacturers may also use a process called hydrogenation to turn unsaturated fat into saturated fat (such as vegetable oil into solid shortening). Whatever form they're in, these are the fats to avoid because they are the number-one dietary culprits in causing high levels of cholesterol and heart disease.

• **Monounsaturated fat.** Monounsaturated fats are the kinds you find in such foods as peanuts, avocados, olives, and oils like olive and canola. You may have heard about the so-called Mediterranean Diet, loaded with these fats and considered to be heart-healthy. While these fats may indeed offer some heart protection (and at least are not *harmful* like saturated fats), they are only needed in small amounts to provide health benefits.

• **Polyunsaturated fat.** Like monounsaturated fat, polyunsaturated fat has been considered heart-healthy, and studies have shown that, when it replaces saturated fat in the diet, it can actually help lower blood cholesterol levels. Foods containing polyunsaturated fat include vegetable oils such as corn, sunflower, safflower, and cottonseed oils; certain soft margarines; and fish such as salmon, mackerel, whitefish, and rainbow trout, which contain omega-3 fatty acids, shown in many studies to help lower blood-cholesterol and triglyceride levels.

Then there's dietary cholesterol. It's not a fat but rather a waxy, fat*like* substance found only in animal products—foods like meat, poultry, fish, whole milk, whole-milk cheeses, and egg yolks. Because dietary cholesterol often contributes to health problems the way excess dietary fat does, it is recommended that you limit your dietary cholesterol to no more than 300 mg per day. (An egg yolk, for example, contains 213 mg, so you see you have to be careful with certain foods.) You'll *also* have to be careful at the supermarket when you see food packages that proudly announce, "No Cholesterol!" without bothering to announce that they *do* contain lots of fat. It simply means that the food has no *animal* fat in it. (We'll talk more about label-reading later.)

We can't make this point strongly enough: A little dietary fat goes a long way. While experts disagree on how much fat is optimal for a healthy diet—recommendations range from as little as 10 to 15 percent (of your daily calorie intake) to the USDA/Department of Health and Human Services suggested 30 percent, with saturated fat comprising no more than 10 percent of your *total fat intake*—most of us are eating too much of the stuff. According to national figures, the average American diet is about 34 percent fat. This means that a person consuming 2,000 calories per day is getting 680 (or 34 percent) of those calories from fat. Remember, every gram of fat, no matter what kind, contains 9 calories. Just one tablespoon of fat is 14 grams, which translates to 126 calories. It adds up fast.

If you're like most people, just reducing your dietary fat by a few percentage points should do much to improve your health. Best of all, it isn't hard to do—and if you follow our plan, you won't have to worry about doing any fancy calculations, either.

What Makes a Healthy Diet?

DECADES OF BAD EATING HABITS—making poor food choices, periods of overeating followed by strict dieting, maybe even cycles of bingeing and purging—may have contributed to your present overweight status. If your eating history sounds anything like this, then it's very possible you don't really know what constitutes a good, healthy diet. But even those of us who consider ourselves pretty smart about healthy eating can use some guidelines. One useful source of healthy-eating information is the U.S. Department of Agriculture and the U.S. Department of Health and Human Services, which every five years updates its *Dietary Guidelines for Americans.* Here is its most current (1995) seven-point plan for healthy eating:

• Eat a variety of foods.

• Balance the food you eat with physical activity—maintain or improve your weight.

• Choose a diet with plenty of grain products, vegetables, and fruit.

• Choose a diet low in fat, saturated fat, and cholesterol.

• Choose a diet moderate in sugars.

• Choose a diet moderate in salt and sodium.

• If you drink alcoholic beverages, do so in moderation.

While governmental agencies are notoriously slow to respond to popular trends, it's nice to see that these new guidelines reflect many of today's realities regarding the public's tastes, habits, and lifestyles. Three notable highlights of the current government guidelines are:

• an acknowledgment that it's okay and indeed healthful to eat a vegetarian diet, if one chooses to. The text says: "Vegetarian diets are consistent with the *Dietary Guidelines for Americans* and can meet Recommended Dietary Allowances for nutrients."

• an acknowledgment that—hey!—food tastes good. The text says: "Eating is one of life's greatest pleasures."

• a recognition of the fact that weight maintenance is for many of us a reasonable health goal. The text says: "Many Americans gain weight, increasing their risk for high blood pressure . . . and other illness. Therefore, most adults should not gain weight."

To these sensible recommendations, we would add the following. We believe a healthy diet should:

• provide a feeling of satiety by providing you with filling foods in reasonable quantities

• prevent feelings of deprivation

• offer as much choice as possible

• include at least some favorite foods each day

• allow for easy weight control (even when weight loss is not possible)

• make you feel good

A bit radical, you say? Perhaps. When was the last time you read a food plan that insisted you feel good while on it or encouraged you to have some of your favorites? Yet it makes perfect sense. How are you going to stick to *any* program, healthy or otherwise, if it *doesn't* make you feel good, if it doesn't let you decide more or less what you're going to eat, and if it doesn't provide at least one or two foods you love each day? And while we're not urging weight loss, we *are* stressing weight control as a reasonable goal for the overweight person. Any sound eating plan should permit you to maintain your weight (or drop some, if you wish) without a struggle.

Creating Your Own Eating Plan

By THIS POINT IN YOUR LIFE (and your weight), you've probably had your fill of programs that tell you what to eat, how much, and when—especially when they didn't give you the desired results. That's why you're going to appreciate the Big Picture Plan. It gives you credit for knowing your body better than anyone else does and for knowing what does and doesn't work for you in terms of eating. In effect, we'll be guiding you through the creation of your own personalized food plan, one that leaves you feeling satisfied, energetic, and comfortable within your own body and helps keep your weight in balance. The goal is to allow you to streamline your eating, whether you cook a lot, eat out a lot, or some combination thereof. By shifting your focus toward the range of healthy foods at your disposal, foods that *you* choose, eating will no longer be the unhealthy or emotionally charged event it may have been throughout your life.

The three keys to the Big Picture Plan for Healthy Eating are these: dietary-fat control, portion control, and food variety.

1. **Dietary-fat control:** Your aim is simple: a gradual cutback on the fat you're presently eating. You are not shooting for a particular number of fat grams per day or a maximum number of high-fat meals per week. Instead, you will start by jotting down your current eating routine for one week, seeing where you stand, more or

less, in terms of your typical intake of high-fat foods. You will then start taking small, manageable steps toward reducing fat for the sake of your health.

2. **Portion control:** At the same time that you're keeping an eye on how much fat you eat, you're going to start becoming more aware of something you may have been ignoring up until now: food *quantity*. That means paying attention to the number and size of the meals and snacks you eat each day. By keeping a conscious-yet-casual watch on your portions, you'll be able to eat many of your favorites in reasonable amounts while at the same time stabilizing your weight and improving your health.

3. **Food variety:** If you strive to eat a wide range of food from the six major categories, you'll never have to worry about whether or not your body is getting all the nutrients it needs; it just automatically will. In a little while, we'll discuss the major food categories and reasonable daily quantities of each.

Like Rolling Off a Log

IT'S IMPOSSIBLE TO CUSTOM-TAILOR a healthy eating plan you can live with for life unless you know how you tend to eat *now*. So, for one week, we suggest that you keep a written log of every morsel of food and drink you put in your mouth, as well as the time of day you have them. Your seven-day food diary may just naturally fall into three main meals plus a series of snacks. Or you may be an all-day "grazer," someone who eats whenever she's hungry or when it's convenient. Or you may tend to skip meals when you're too rushed to eat, and then make up for it later in the day. Or you may be a meal-skipper in the belief that it's a good way to control your weight. (It isn't.)

Whatever your pattern happens to be, just jot it all down for seven full days to see how often and how much you tend to eat, and what your food favorites are. After this first week of inventory-taking, you need not continue to keep a written food log unless you want to.

How to Cut the Fat (So You Hardly Feel It)

WE SAID IT BEFORE: You're going to make small, easy changes in your diet so that eating remains the pleasurable experience it should be. Remember: Gradual change leads to permanent changes. Here are some key ways to effect those subtle yet powerful changes:

• **Make a qualitative change in your menu.** Now that you've kept a week-long food log, what does it reveal to you? Are you eating a lot of cheese, chocolate, or other fatty foods? Are you eating meat at most dinners? Using this log will show you how to make simple qualitative changes in your eating. For instance, if you were to decide to eat just one extra vegetable and one extra piece of fruit each day, you would probably displace some fatty foods from your diet, and as a result, your overall fat consumption would automatically be lower.

Or your goal might be to reduce the number of red-meat meals you eat each week from, say, five this week to four for the next two weeks, to three for the following two weeks, and maybe just one or two the week after that. The substitutes? Fish, skinless chicken, beans, tofu, and other lower-fat protein products. By the end of that period, it's likely that you won't even miss the meat.

Trying to record and adhere to a daily fat-gram quota is silly—and unnecessary. You can attempt to do the calculations, but if you're like most of us, maybe you'll do them once or twice. (How many people do you know who count fat grams or calories on a daily basis?) Take the pressure off yourself and work on making *qualitative* eating changes instead of quantitative ones.

• **Strike a healthy balance.** As we've said before, cutting fat doesn't mean cutting *out* fat completely. Just learn to balance your low-fat foods with your not-so-low-fat foods. Yes, you *can* occasionally eat pizza as long as you balance it over the week with other low-fat foods. By becoming more alert to what you're choosing and by making a real effort to balance your foods, you'll probably automatically lower your fat intake to a nice 25 to 30 percent range. In time, if you're consistent in your dietary changes, you'll get to the point where you've significantly lowered your fat intake, and should you want that occasional ice cream sundae or piece of cheesecake, you can eat it without harm. Your body won't notice a rare fat-loading because, on balance, you're eating a low-fat diet overall.

• **Swap your high-fat favorites for low-fat favorites.** To improve your diet, you may need to move from the food you *love* to the food you *like*. And that may simply mean finding low-fat versions of your favorites.

If you're a chocoholic, drink fat-free cocoa or have an occasional fat-free brownie. Love snack foods? Guiltless Gourmet and Frito-Lay both make delicious baked, no-fat chips you can have with salsa. Alpine Lace has a line of tasty lower-fat cheeses. There are many excellent choices out there so that you can eat very well and not feel deprived. (And along the way, you may find what many of us have already discovered: once you significantly reduce the fat in your diet, you simply cannot eat the quantities of high-fat foods you ate before without feeling uncomfortable and engorged very quickly.)

Here are 11 other easy swaps you can make:

1. **margarine:** try spreading your bagel or toast with fat-free cream cheese or all-fruit spread
2. **whole milk:** try drinking 1 percent milk, skim milk or the new skim milk with added milk solids
3. **shortening:** try cooking with a nonfat cooking spray, wine or broth, or a small amount of olive oil
4. **mayonnaise and salad dressing:** try fat-free mayo and dressings, or sprinkle your salad with lots of fresh herbs, lemon, balsamic vinegar, or flavored vinegars
5. **American cheese:** try making your sandwich with fat-free cheese
6. **ground beef:** try preparing your burger or meat loaf using ground turkey or veal or extra-lean beef

7. **low-fat milk:** try lowering the fat further still with skim or 1 percent milk

8. **eggs:** try making your scrambled eggs or omelets with fat-free egg substitutes, or just use the egg whites

9. **butter:** try butter substitutes or salsa atop your vegetables or baked potato

10. **ice cream:** try fat-free frozen desserts, frozen yogurt, sorbet, or fresh fruit

11. **pork sausage:** try turkey sausage

• **Eat the fat-free stuff first.** Fill up on fresh fruits and vegetables (including the "Five a Day" servings of produce recommended by the National Cancer Institute for optimum health), grains, breads, pasta, beans, and rice, and you won't be as hungry for—or tempted by—the more fattening alternatives. Remember, the more you choose the fat-free foods, the more you're automatically displacing some of the high-fat stuff. For instance, if you're in a restaurant and you order a fresh-fruit cup as an appetizer, chances are you'll eat less of the beef stroganoff *and* you may be too full to order the chocolate mousse that tempted you when you first spied it on the menu.

• **Give low-fat a chance.** The thought of cutting fat (a little or completely) from high-fat foods may make your heart sink, but it's not as bad as you may imagine. Many people who start to make these kinds of dietary changes report that the less fat they eat, the less they crave it and the more they enjoy the taste and texture of nonfat foods. Don't be surprised if, one day, you pick up some plain, raw radishes or cherry tomatoes, crunch on them, and decide, Hey, these taste pretty good! Sure, bread and butter tastes wonderful, but warm-from-the-oven Italian bread *without* any fat on it has an enjoyable flavor all its own. Give yourself a chance to appreciate the taste of delicious foods minus the fat (or with less of it).

• **Spark the flavor.** How do you get over your resistance to eating low-fat foods? By making them taste good! Here are some quick-

and-easy ways to add zip to your low-fat meals:

• Cook foods in nonfat cooking spray, fat-free consommé, wine, or juice instead of butter or oil.

• Season your foods with a variety of fresh herbs and spices. Garlic, curry powder, grated lemon and orange peel, and even raisins are great ways to add lots of flavor without fat.

• Use your microwave to prepare vegetables with plenty of color and crunch and practically no loss of vitamins.

• Use applesauce or pureed prunes in cake recipes instead of shortening or butter.

• In low-fat recipes calling for nonfat yogurt, you may want to add a bit of low-fat ricotta cheese for extra body and sweetness.

Bookstores are packed with cookbooks aimed at today's health-conscious chef. Three excellent examples: *500 Fat-Free Recipes* by Sarah Schlesinger (Villard); *The Light Touch Cookbook* by Marie Simmons (Chapters); and *Cooking for Good Health* by Gloria Rose (Avery).

• **Be a savvy shopper.** For most of us, healthy eating begins in the supermarket. Once you stop worrying about whether what you're eating will lead to weight loss, your main dietary challenge is to discipline yourself to shop differently and to prepare food in a low-fat manner for the sake of weight maintenance and your general health. If your shopping list used to be packed with high-fat items, just make up a new one filled with tasty, low-fat substitutes, following the guidelines above, plus any others you wish to add. As we've said before, these changes don't have to be radical; slow and steady will get you where you want to go.

Here are four more smart shopping tips:

1. **Learn to read and understand the Nutrition Facts labels on food packages.** They will help you distinguish the low-fat foods (with under 5 grams of fat per serving, such as most breads, fresh fruits and vegetables, low-fat meats and poultry, and low-fat salad dressings) from the medium-fat foods (with up to 10 grams of fat per serving, including certain frozen entrees, whole-fat cheeses, bacon, packaged croissants and muffins, and certain chips) from the

high-fat foods (with 11 or more grams of fat per serving, including peanut butter, packaged cakes, nuts, ice cream, packaged breaded chicken, and hot dogs).

Two important points to be aware of when reading these labels: 1) the nutrition breakdowns are *per serving*, not per package, so you must check to see how many servings are in the package; and 2) the Percentage Daily Value (that is, how much of your total nutrient requirements are satisfied by this food) is based on a 2,000- to 2,500-calorie daily diet. If you're eating less than that (which most women probably are), then you've got to scale down the percentages accordingly.

2. **Don't shop when you're hungry.** If you're ravenous, you'll be likelier to make impulse buys that aren't wise.

3. **Learn the layout of your favorite supermarket.** You'll get used to heading straight for the low-fat aisles (fresh produce, canned beans and vegetables, breads, rice and pasta, low-fat dairy products) and zigzag around the other aisles packed with high-fat land mines.

4. **Buy the best, freshest foods you can afford.** You'll never miss the taste of fatty foods if you select sweet, luscious fruits from the farmer's market or local greenmarket, pungent spices and herbs from ethnic shops, or just-baked bread from the bakery.

• **Eat with your eyes—and your taste buds—open.** We never told you *not* to eat an occasional cheese omelet or ice cream cone, but when you do, eat it with awareness *and* with gusto! You'll discover that, when you do have it, you'll enjoy it all the more *and* you probably won't eat as much of it. Sometimes, one tiny piece of Godiva chocolate is actually more soul-satisfying than a whole quart of low-fat chocolate frozen yogurt.

• **Remind yourself why you're doing this!** Whenever we seek pleasure without thought of giving our body what it needs, sooner or later that spells trouble. Sure, you'll never mistake a banana for a pint of Häagen-Dazs, but you'll feel *much* better after eating the fruit. It really helps to have a certain amount of discipline and rationality in your lifestyle, and it's smart to be aware of the long-term consequences of your immediate actions. In a sense, you're investing in your future health by passing up that pecan pie or that Big Mac. Consider giving up a little something today so you'll be a lot better off tomorrow.

• **Low-fat's great, but** . . . Keep things in perspective—including the benefits of switching to a lower-fat diet. Yes, it's important, but reducing your fat intake isn't a magic bullet for your health. If you cut your dietary fat but you smoke, you're sedentary, and you don't manage your stress, you're still at high risk for ill health. Health is promoted through a change of a *number* of behaviors, not just one.

Portion Alert!

CUTTING FAT IS ALL WELL AND GOOD, and thanks to the overwhelming availability of such wonderful things as Famous Amos fat-free brownies, Guiltless Gourmet fat-free chips, Wish-Bone fat-free bleu-cheese dressing and Ben & Jerry's fat-free frozen yogurt, we Americans *have* been cutting back on our fat intake. Hmmm . . . Then why has our national obesity rate risen from 25 to about 30 percent in the past 15 years or so? A safe bet would be that we're probably not exercising as much as we should *and* we're eating too much (albeit healthier) food.

Using lower-fat foods to replace the higher-fat ones we love is an excellent way to cut fat *and* cut calories—as long as we *don't* compensate for the calorie savings by eating twice as much of the healthy stuff! To keep your weight from going up further and to avoid health problems associated with increasing weight, you've got to be as aware of your serving sizes and frequency of eating as you are of your fat intake.

If you shoot for three reasonable-size meals plus two to three healthy snacks per day, or some variation on that, you should do fine. (If you're a diabetic, you may need more frequent smaller meals to keep your blood sugar levels in check.) Here is a list of what constitutes **one serving** for each of the major food categories:

Grain Products (bread, cereal, rice, and pasta)

- 1 slice of bread
- 1 oz. ready-to-eat cereal
- ½ cup cooked cereal, rice, or pasta

Vegetables

- 1 cup raw leafy vegetables
- ½ cup other types of vegetables (cooked or chopped raw)
- ¾ cup vegetable juice

Fruits

- 1 medium apple, banana, orange, etc.
- ½ cup chopped, cooked, or canned fruit
- ¾ cup fruit juice

Milk Products (milk, yogurt, and cheese)

- 1 cup milk or yogurt
- 1½ oz. whole-milk cheese
- 2 oz. processed cheese (low-fat or fat-free)

Meat and Beans (meat, poultry, fish, dried beans, eggs, and nuts)

- 2-3 oz. cooked lean meat, poultry, or fish
- ½ cup cooked dried beans = 1 oz. lean meat
- 1 egg = 1 oz. lean meat
- 2 Tbsp. peanut butter = 1 oz. meat
- ⅓ cup nuts = 1 oz. meat

The USDA/Department of Health and Human Services has turned these five food groups—along with Fats/Oils/Sweets, a sixth group to be used "sparingly"—into the Food Guide Pyramid, which you've probably seen by now on bags of bread, boxes of cereal, and other food packages. Here are the **recommended number of daily servings** for each food group:

Grain Products: 6-11 servings
Vegetables: 3-5 servings
Fruits: 2-4 servings
Milk Products: 2-3 servings
Meat and Beans, etc.: 2-3 servings

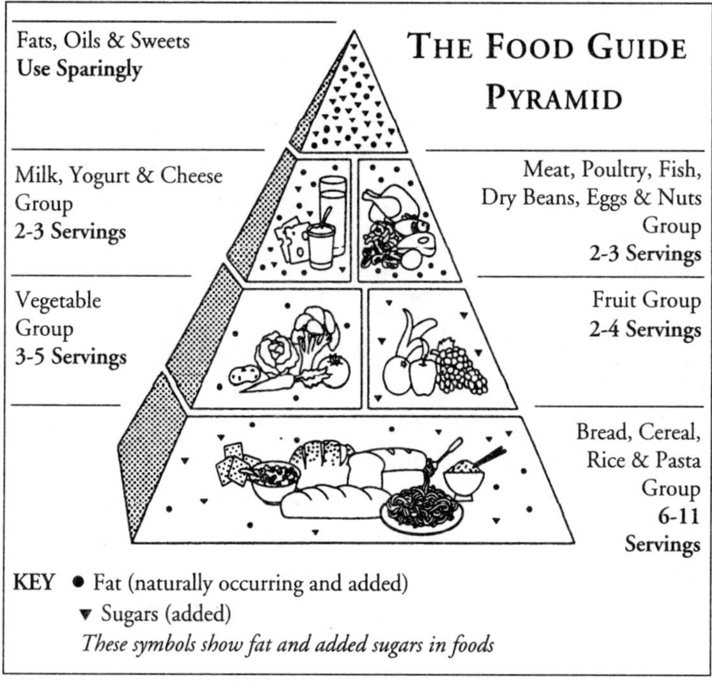

Source: U.S. Department of Agriculture/U.S. Department of Health and Human Services

Even if you were to stick to the high-end number of these servings each day, you should not find yourself gaining weight, particularly if you exercise regularly. (More on exercise in the next chapter.) In fact, you may well find yourself slowly and gradually *losing* some weight, especially if these servings are fewer than you've been used to.

Although we've said that we don't want you to become a fanatic about weighing and measuring your food or counting your calories, it *is* important to be able to know pretty much at a glance whether you're looking at one, three or six servings of food on your plate, particularly when you're eating out. For example, some restaurants serve massive portions—16-ounce steaks, three cups of pasta, huge slabs of cheesecake—in order to keep customers coming back for more. (And who among us *doesn't* like to feel as though we got our money's worth when we eat out?)

The problem is that, in our effort to maintain our membership in the Clean Plate Club, we tend to eat much more than is good for us. Which is why it's vital to get into the healthy habit of accurately judging (give or take an ounce or two) sensible portion sizes. Practicing at home while cooking is the easiest way to get the hang of it. You can also use these convenient little measuring techniques using your own hand:

- 1 ounce of small snack foods (like peanuts) is equal to one handful
- 1 ounce of larger snack foods (like chips) is equal to two handfuls
- 1 teaspoon of peanut butter, mayonnaise, etc. is equal in size to the top joint of your thumb
- 1 ounce of cheese is equal in size to your whole thumb
- 3 ounces of meat, poultry, or fish is equal in size to your palm *without* thumb and fingers
- 1 cup of pasta, rice, cereal, etc. is equal in size to your closed fist

Sugars/Salt & Sodium/Alcohol

MODERATION IN ALL THINGS: You've heard it before and it's certainly a philosophy to which we subscribe, particularly where it comes to food. We've already discussed how dietary fat, for all its good taste, should be used in moderation in order to prevent or ease health problems. The same holds true for those fun "extras" that help to make many of our meals so yummy—but often lead to health woes.

For example, refined sugar, such as table sugar, tastes good and is relatively low in calories (18 per teaspoon). But those are empty calories—that is, they provide little in the way of nutrition. Furthermore, excess sugar has been found to be a culprit in such other health problems as dental caries, increased triglyceride levels, decreased calcium absorption, fatigue, and irritability. In addition, many of our food favorites that are high in sugar are *also* high in fat, causing a double whammy to our health. So sugar should be used sparingly. If you're a sugar fan, you can gradually wean yourself off high quantities of the sweet stuff using the same method we described for cutting back on fat—by slowly reducing the number of high-sugar foods and snacks you eat. In time, you will probably lose your taste for overly sweet, sugary foods.

Sodium and salt should also be used in moderation because they can cause high blood pressure. Healthy people are urged to limit their sodium intake to no more than 3,000 mg a day—the equivalent of a mere 1½ teaspoons of salt. If you're one of those folks who routinely sprinkles salt onto your food before you've even tasted it, now's the time to start thinking twice before you automatically reach for the salt shaker, and maybe experiment with some sodium-free salt substitutes. Even if you don't normally add a lot of salt to your food, you've still got to keep an eye on other sources of sodium. Some of those high-sodium culprits are obvious—heavily salted chips and similar salty snack foods, for instance. But others, such as pickles, low-calorie frozen entrees, and even super-healthy canned beans and certain ready-to-eat cereals, are packed with sodium. If you aren't careful, you can easily consume in one sitting two or more times the sodium that would be the maximum for an entire day.

As for alcohol, many folks consider it the ideal way to "unwind" after a hard day at the office, or they may regard a glass of fine wine as the perfect accompaniment to a good meal. No one's saying that you've got to eliminate alcohol from your healthy eating plan. Indeed, some studies show that there may be some heart-protective benefits to be derived from drinking a modest amount of wine each day. So, again, think moderation. In excess, alcohol increases your risk for a whole host of serious problems, including high blood pressure, stroke, heart disease, certain cancers, birth defects, and damage to the brain, liver, and pancreas—not to mention drinking-related automobile and other accidents and risks to your personal relationships. If you do drink, limit it to one a day if you're a woman and two a day if you're a man. (One drink consists of 12 ounces of regular beer, 5 ounces of wine or 1.5 ounces of 80-proof distilled spirits.)

Variety for Good Nutrition

As we stressed before, a *variety* of good, nutritious, low-fat foods will virtually guarantee a healthy diet. Making sure you build plenty of your favorite foods into your food plan will also ensure that you'll stick with it, week after week, month after month. Check back to your original seven-day food log. Now that you have a sense of what adjustments you'll need to make in terms of cutting fat and possibly reducing portion sizes, are you *also* getting a good variety of foods from the five main food groups? If you feel you'd still like a little guidance in terms of following a sound food plan that provides plenty of variety, you can try a sensible commercial food program, such as Weight Watchers, or Richard Simmons's Deal-A-Meal, which is available in many department and discount stores. Although these are ostensibly weight-loss food plans, because they are all sensible and nutritious, you can use them to assure yourself that you're taking in a variety of healthy foods each day. Or you can order one of the following publications: *The Food Guide Pyramid: Your Personal Guide to Healthful Eating* or the 1995 edition of *Nutrition and Your Health: Dietary Guidelines for Americans*, which includes the Food Guide Pyramid. (See Resources, page 245, for ordering information.)

Do You Need Vitamin Supplements?

A visit to your local health-food store or pharmacy is all it should take to convince you that vitamin and mineral supplements are big business. And if you listen to television and radio commercials and read magazine ads for nutrition supplements, you might easily conclude that there's surely *some* supplement out there meant for *you*—whether it's one promising to give you more energy, help ward off cancer, or slow the aging process.

Yet not all supplements deliver what their promotional ads say they do. For example, *no* vitamin pill can give you more energy; only calories can do that. Even taking nutritional supplements from the most reputable manufacturers (and there are a few) isn't nearly as good as the nutrients you get from the very best source—namely, healthy *food.* The iron you might ingest from a pill can't hold a candle to the iron you'd get from a simple cup of Cream of Wheat, and the cancer-fighting beta-carotene found in a fresh carrot or sweet potato puts a beta-carotene supplement to shame. When you know that a good, well-balanced diet, such as that prescribed by the Food Guide Pyramid (page 115), gives you all the nutrients your body needs to stay healthy, why would you ever want to spend extra money on supplements? For the vast majority of healthy people who eat right, they are unnecessary.

There are some exceptions, of course. For instance, if you believe that, for whatever reason, you probably don't eat a healthy, varied diet most days of the week, then you might want to take a one-a-day-type multivitamin for insurance. You might be urged by your health-care provider to take supplements if you've been diagnosed with a particular problem that can be eased or eliminated with supplementation—for example, iron pills for iron-deficiency anemia. And many women are urged by their doctors to take calcium supplements because the calcium found even in most healthy food plans may not be enough to help prevent osteoporosis. You may want to discuss your questions about supplements with your health-care professional.

Water, Water Everywhere . . .

WHEN YOU REALIZE THAT OUR BODIES are more than half water—it makes up 80 percent of our blood, 70 percent of our brain and even 20 percent of our bones—it's easy to see why we're always being urged to drink those six to eight glasses a day. Water is vital for all body functions, from digestion to the delivery of nutrients throughout our body to the elimination of wastes. Water helps keep our skin smooth and supple. What's more, drinking some water before and in between meals provides a nice feeling of fullness, which may help prevent overeating.

For some folks, the idea of drinking all that water each day is intimidating. But keep in mind that your water requirement can be met by drinking a combination of tap or bottled water, seltzer, club soda, diet soda, or herbal tea. Do *not* include caffeinated drinks, such as coffee or colas, toward fulfilling your water quota—these are diuretics and, if anything, will cause you to excrete even more liquid than you took in by drinking them.

Many people—particularly those who have been on and off diets for much of their lives—report that they've lost their ability to identify real hunger, and often what they believe are hunger pangs is actually the sensation of thirst. Try this experiment: The next time you think you're hungry and "shouldn't" be—because you recently ate a good-size meal, for example—drink a glass of water instead of reaching for a snack. You may be pleasantly surprised to find that the water was exactly what your body was craving.

The End of Emotional Eating

AFTER YEARS AND YEARS of being told how, when, what, and how much to eat (and *not* to eat), you may well have approached this chapter with trepidation. As we've indicated from the beginning of this book, we understand the frustration you've no doubt experienced with your weight and the various eating programs you may have tried since becoming a large-size person. But we want you to feel the sense of satisfaction and relief that comes with viewing food as a means to nourish your body and help you become healthier—not as The Enemy.

We know it won't be easy for some of you. After what may be a lifetime of developing powerful emotional issues around food, it may take a while before you can actually sit down and enjoy a healthy, sensible meal without all the worry associated with how it may or may not affect your weight. But that's why this book, and in particular this chapter, was written: to help you gradually learn to use food for its intended positive purpose—not as an emotional crutch, a balm for bad feelings, or a weapon of self-destruction. Perhaps for the first time ever, you're hearing people tell you to stop obsessing about your weight and start thinking about your health, your longevity, and your acceptance of your current weight. We sincerely hope that you can, at long last, put food in its rightful place in your life—and get on with the rest of your life.

PROFILE

Debra Davidson

New York, New York
Age: 41
Height: 5'7"
Weight: 200 pounds
Occupation: Marketing executive

AS A TEENAGER, I was always about 20 pounds overweight. Then I started dieting. Initially, I lost the weight I wanted to lose, but then it went skyrocketing back up, with an extra 25 pounds added on top of that. That was the beginning of my up-and-down weight and compulsive-eating behavior. Since then, my weight has been in the 150-to-200-pound range, stabilizing at around 180 to 200 in the last few years. Still, I don't consider my weight a real problem. Now I'm about 200 pounds and a size 16, but I'm fairly tall and I believe I look thinner than I am. I dress very well, and I'm always well groomed, and my weight is definitely not the first thing people see when I walk into a room.

I was married for seven years, and at my wedding, I weighed around 160 pounds. My husband was quite accepting of me in any shape or form, but I was dissatisfied with myself, and so I was angry and depressed a lot of the time. I can honestly say that our divorce eight years ago had nothing to do with my husband's feelings about my weight.

Since then, I've been dating whenever I can. Over the years, I've placed three personal ads, and the last time I did it, I decided to take a chance and reveal my weight. Why? Well, I wasn't about to describe myself as thin and fit, which is what 99 percent of people say in their ads, whether it's true or not. Also,

Profile

I didn't want to have to deal with the issue over the phone; I wanted to preempt it. Of the three ads I've placed, this last one got the smallest response—only about 10 letters, and none of them very promising. I really don't know how much of it had to do with my size, or even with my age. It would be interesting to run the same exact ad without mentioning my weight, as a control, and see what happens. Despite this experience, I'm optimistic about my chances of meeting nice men, and I hope to remarry someday.

If you had asked me seven or eight years ago if I thought my weight affected my social life, I would have said yes, that it definitely put me out of the running with certain men. But today, I think there are many other factors—I know many women who are thin and don't date any more than I do. Although I'm much heavier now than, say, when I was married, I feel lighter! I think that's because I have a better self-image.

Psychotherapy has helped me become comfortable with my body. A lot of times in the past, I believed it was the weight that was bothering me. But through therapy, I've come to understand that it was something else. Weight was always easier to blame than the real issue—which is not to say that, if I could snap my fingers and be 20 or 30 pounds thinner, I wouldn't; of course I would, if I knew it would be permanent. It's easier to live as a thinner person. I'm fairly vain, and I love to have a lot of choices when I'm out buying clothes, and I don't like to have to think twice before choosing a seat on the bus, and these things wouldn't be such issues if I were thinner. I also don't like the idea that some people still associate being overweight with being undisciplined, lazy, slovenly, and underachieving. It's not true in my case; I do quite well in my job. Nor does my weight affect my health very much. While I may get fatigued more easily than thinner people, my blood pressure is low, and I'm generally healthy.

Profile

Although today I can accept my weight, I would say that dieting has probably hurt me more than anything else. If I hadn't been so driven as a teenager to lose those 20 or 25 pounds—if I had just accepted my weight and kept eating as I did—I might have gained more weight, but I bet I'd be a lot smaller today than I am. I probably also wouldn't have developed the bad eating habits I still have. I have friends who are parents, and they're concerned about the way their children eat, particularly their daughters. I'm very outspoken when these friends attempt to control their children's eating habits. Even if these kids eat excessively at times, I feel that if they're deprived of certain foods, they'll be more likely to obsess about them and possibly develop bad habits, the way I did.

While I continue to work on eating more healthfully, I've learned that it's important to really accept yourself, to take ownership of your body and to accept it just as you would, for example, a less-than-perfect nose. Even if your body isn't considered ideal by society's standards, accept that you have this body and love yourself in spite of it. Then, take whatever steps you need to take to improve your behavior. Make self-improvement, not perfection, your goal.

PROFILE

Kathy Devine

Menomonee Falls, Wisconsin
Age: 39
Height: 5'10"
Weight: 325 pounds ("the last time I checked")
Occupation: Hospital reception supervisor

I PROBABLY LOOKED LIKE ANY OTHER KID until I got to third or fourth grade, when I started getting pudgy. From there, I just got bigger and bigger. My parents are also overweight (although I'm the biggest in the family), so I think it must be a genetic thing with me. In fact, now my son, Sean, is in third grade and I see *him* starting to look a little pudgy, the way I did at his age. Having grown up overweight and lived through the teasing, I don't want Sean to go through that. He tells me he hasn't been teased yet, but I think it's out there, and I worry about it a little bit. As for me and my weight, it's no big deal to him. In fact, he wants to show me off—he's always begging me to chaperone his class's field trips. Sean never acts ashamed of me or tries to hide me from his friends. His mom is soft and cuddly, and that's all he's ever known. He adores me the way I am.

The same is true of my husband, Patrick. He loves me. He's definitely a fat admirer—he *loves* large, round women. We met through a personal ad he placed in *Big Beautiful Woman* magazine. I answered it, and we hit it off right away. When I was young and single, I hated my butt and my thighs, and I thought, I'll never meet anybody, looking this way. But Pat loved my shape, and for once, I wasn't embarrassed or unhappy about the way I am. To him, I'm the most perfect thing, and that's what it's all about: finding that one person who loves

PROFILE

everything about you, even the things you don't like about yourself. That's how I knew Pat was the right guy for me. In fact, every now and then I'll catch him ogling some big woman on the street—the way other men might stare at a thin blonde. So I *know* he's sincere about loving me the way I am. Pat makes me feel beautiful. I've even asked him, "What if I got sick and I *lost* a lot of weight? Would you still love me if I were thin?" Of course, he says yes!

How did I come to terms with my weight? I've done my share of dieting, along with everyone else in America, and after a while, it became obvious that I was never going to go from 325 pounds to 125 pounds. When I see other people obsessing about their weight, I think, Doesn't it dawn on you that this is how you're probably going to be? So much of it has to do with genetics, so are you going to be depressed for the rest of your life or get on with it?

It's important to get support for who you are. I'm so lucky to have found the man of my dreams, but he's not the only one—there are others out there who like big women. You just have to go out and find them. If you don't have a romantic partner who's supportive, at least find a friend who is. I've talked about my weight with my thinner friends, and they say, "We don't look at you as being fat; we look at you as being *you*, Kathy." None of my friends is ashamed to be with me because I'm fat. You need to find people like that, people for whom your weight is not an issue. Or join an organization like NAAFA [National Association to Advance Fat Acceptance]. NAAFA has been great for me—they're very supportive. You don't know what it's like until you're in a room full of people where, for once, you're not the biggest one there. I wish more young people would get involved in this kind of outreach. It's so important to connect with people who are big and *living*—not hiding out.

PROFILE

I don't eat huge quantities of food. My husband is thin, and we eat the same meal every night—*and* we have our share of leftovers at the end of the meal. Maybe I'm not watching the fat count of everything that goes in my mouth, and when someone else is having a rice cake, I may be eating potato chips, but it'll be a few chips, not an entire bag, the way I think most people might expect. I think I eat pretty much like an average person. For example, right now in my office, I have a banana, a bag of rice cakes, and a NutriGrain bar. For breakfast today, I had some yogurt and a NutriGrain bar. Most of the time, I really watch and plan what I eat. I may, for instance, have a salad one day for lunch when I know I'm going to have enchiladas for dinner, but that's what thin people do. Sure, sometimes someone will bring in some brownies to work and I'll grab one. It happens. I'm just doing the day-to-day living everyone else is doing. Some meals you watch, and some you don't. By doing that, I find that my weight stays about the same.

While I'm not making efforts to lose weight, I *am* making efforts to stay in shape. I have a CardioGlide at home, and I use it a minimum of three times a week. The CardioGlide helps me stretch and feel better. I try to do a few sit-ups when I wake up in the morning, and I also do a lot of walking. And I *love* gardening—we have a big yard, and in the summer, we're outside all the time. You need to do things to help keep your legs and heart strong.

Accepting yourself is a mindset—you've got to find your own inner peace. I always joke, "In my next life, I'm coming back as a thin person, but in *this* life, this is how I am!" Getting thin is every fat person's dream, but the question is, How do you do it and *stay* there without suffering? Is being thin that big a deal? I know that if I had to live on rice cakes to stay thin, I'd be the biggest crab!

CHAPTER SIX

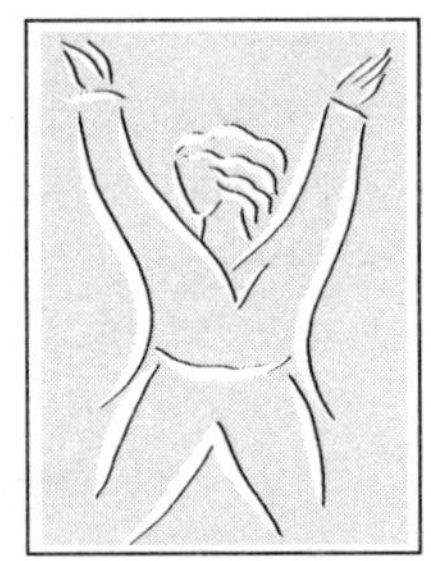

THE BIG PICTURE PLAN *for* HEALTH:

Exercise

IN THE PREVIOUS CHAPTER, we talked about how years and years of dieting and unsuccessful weight-loss attempts may have made you understandably gun-shy about following *any* food plan, healthy or otherwise. For the same reasons, you may be exercise-phobic, someone who sees a person on a treadmill or power-walking through the park and thinks, Been there, done that. Thanks, but that's definitely *not* for me. If D-I-E-T is a four-letter word in your mind, then maybe the eight-letter word E-X-E-R-C-I-S-E seems *twice* as bad.

Whether you're obese, slender, or somewhere in between, you can always come up with an excuse not to exercise—and, regrettably, millions of Americans do. A three-year study called "What We Eat in America," being conducted by the Beltsville Human Nutrition Research Center in Riverdale, Maryland, reveals that in 1995, 27 percent of men and 43 percent of women admitted that they "rarely" engaged in vigorous physical activity. And the U.S. Public

Health Service reports that only about 20 percent of adults exercise regularly. So if you're physically inactive (or close to it), you've got plenty of company.

Why are so many of us sedentary? Mostly because "progress" has made it a cinch to sit back and relax while doing those things our fathers and mothers used to strain to do. Today, you can "ride" a lawnmower, wash and dry clothes at the push of a button, and make bread in an electric bread-maker. It's almost as though the barons of the Industrial Revolution conspired to make us a country of lazybones by taking all the work out of daily living. While none of us wants to return to a world without television channel changers or frost-free refrigerators, there's no denying that all this push-button technology has taken a toll on our national health. And there's only one way to combat a sedentary lifestyle—exercise.

Many of us have told ourselves countless times throughout our lives, "Today's the day I'm going to start exercising!" But the question is: Are we *still* exercising now? And are we doing it several days each week, the way it was meant to be done—and the only way it can do us any good? The fact is, launching a serious exercise program takes real commitment. Unlike improving your diet or quitting smoking, engaging in regular exercise is a health-promotion activity that requires an ongoing commitment of *time*—not just this week, not just this month, but *forever*. And we can hear you saying, "Hey, in my busy life, who has time to work out three times a week . . . forever?"

Well, for that matter, do we have time to floss our teeth every single morning or buckle up our seat belts each time we get behind the wheel or replace the batteries in our smoke detectors every six months or spend a few extra minutes at the market whenever we shop, really reading those package labels to make sure we're getting nutritious food? Yet, busy though we are, we who do these things somehow manage to *make* the time because we've decided that our health and our longevity are worth it. And exercise is right up there in the pantheon of health activities that are worth every moment you spend doing them, however much or little time that may be.

Which leads us to what may be the best possible news about exercise: that you need not commit hours and hours of time each week to derive some health benefit. Even if you're a card-carrying couch potato today, adding a mere 30 minutes a day a few days a week of blood-pumping activity to your life will lengthen and improve the quality of that life. You may have heard about the classic studies claiming that unless you get your heart rate up to a certain aerobic level and unless you exercise for extended periods of time, you will derive little or no benefit. But more recent studies have shown that even moderate exercise on a regular basis does confer certain health benefits and will definitely help you feel better—*and* better about yourself. If you can't manage much more than a *little* more exercise each week than you're doing now, that's okay. For if you do it *consistently*, you will reap benefits that you will feel almost immediately. We promise.

And here's something else to consider while you're worrying about how you're going to find the time to exercise: Many people report that a regular workout several days a week (or more) actually *adds* time to their day. How is that possible? By making them feel better and more energetic and thereby giving them additional *productive* time. Remember, it's not how many hours a day you have but how *effectively* you use them.

The Health Benefits of Regular Exercise

EXERCISE HAS ALWAYS BEEN CONSIDERED a key component of weight control. And regular workouts *do* help some people lose weight and maintain that weight loss long-term. But whether or not your past exercise efforts have produced similar results for you, we're now talking about the value of exercise for your *health* and *well-being*, regardless of your current weight and regardless of your weight-related goals. We'll repeat a point we made in the last chapter: When you follow a healthy program for its own sake—rather than for how much weight it may or may not help you lose—

that activity becomes so much more enjoyable and pressure-free. Once you get into the groove of swimming a few mornings a week or going for an after-dinner walk because you've discovered it can be *fun* and because you appreciate what it's doing for your overall health—not because you're hoping to lose 10 pounds by the end of the month—chances are you'll like it even more and stick with it indefinitely.

What are the non-weight-related health benefits of exercise? There are many:

- It tones your muscles, making your body feel firmer and look better.
- It increases your level of "good" HDL cholesterol, which, in turn, helps you lower your overall cholesterol reading.
- It increases the efficiency of your heart and lungs.
- Aerobic exercise (more about this later) can help protect against heart disease later in life.
- It may increase your life expectancy.
- It may lower your blood pressure.
- It helps build stronger bones, thus protecting against osteoporosis.
- It may improve the quality of your sleep and ease or eliminate insomnia.
- It may help you to think more clearly.
- It reduces stress, anxiety and/or depression.
- It improves self-esteem and helps create a more positive attitude.
- If you're older, it can help you maintain your functional independence.
- It may improve your sex life.
- If you exercise with others, it helps build and/or enhance your social relationships.

Although regular exercise may not produce weight *loss* for you, it will definitely help you to *maintain* your present weight more easily. Another nice plus: It will probably allow you to eat more food, if you want to, without causing weight gain.

Since you know you have to devote time to it—and since you may not be a big exercise fan to begin with—then we know that you've *really* got to be convinced of its value. We're certain that there must be at least a couple of items on the above list that you'd like to see happen in your life. Regular exercise can help you reach many health goals, possibly better than any other single activity can.

Why Do You Hate to Exercise?

THERE ARE EXCEPTIONS, of course, but it seems as if the majority of large-size people don't like exercise very much. Your reasons can range from not feeling as though you can "keep up" to not liking the way your body looks in exercise clothes to fearing the stares or comments from slimmer folks who might be watching you ride your bike or work out on the StairMaster at the gym. Maybe, for one reason or another, you grew frustrated with your previous workout routine, or maybe when you tried to exercise in the past, you injured yourself. Or, quite possibly, you simply can't imagine an exercise routine you'd enjoy—not for any length of time, anyway.

Many of these complaints are perfectly legitimate. Still, we believe that we can (gently) counter every single one of your possible objections:

• **Can't keep up with others?** Remember, you're not in competition with anyone, not even with yourself. If you go at a pace that's comfortable for *you*, your exercise program will be challenging but doable. Later in this chapter, we'll outline a sensible schedule that you can adapt to your capabilities, going at your own pace.

• **Don't like how your body looks in exercise clothes or don't want to exercise in front of others?** Then don't! You needn't leave your bedroom or basement to do your workout, not with the wide range of home-fitness devices (many of which are foldable for storage and take up very little room when not in use) and exercise videos available. Embarrassed to go outside to walk? Walk on a treadmill at home. Hate the thought of going to the pool to swim or do water exercises? Try at-home step aerobics instead. Lots of people have success with at-home workout programs they've created for themselves.

• **Are you a frustrated former exerciser?** It's very possible that your frustration stems from the fact that you tried exercise specifically to try to lose weight, but it didn't work for you. Put that experience behind you. Now you're no longer exercising for weight loss but rather for *health.* So stop worrying about what the scale says after that workout and just do it for its own sake. If a particular sport or activity no longer interests you, now's the ideal time to try something new.

• **Injured yourself in the past?** Perhaps you weren't exercising properly or safely. Maybe you tried to do too much too soon. Assuming your injury has had sufficient time to heal, you're probably ready to try again! But this time, *ease* into it. If all you think you can manage right now is to work out two days a week, for 15 minutes at a time, that's fine. You can always reevaluate your program down the road. (And later, we'll show you exercise techniques that will help you prevent future injuries.)

• **Don't think there's any exercise you'd enjoy doing?** You're not using your imagination! We have plenty of suggestions throughout this chapter that will help you expand your definition of "exercise" and let you see the myriad choices you have. One or more is sure to be fun for *you.*

What's the Best Exercise for You?

PEOPLE ASK US ALL THE TIME: "What exercise should *I* be doing?" "Which exercise will give *me* the best results?"

Whenever we hear that question, our answer is invariably: The best exercise for you is the one (or more, done in rotation) that keeps you exercising on a regular basis. In fact, it doesn't matter *which* activity you select, as long as it gets your heart rate up some, gets you to do some sweating, and keeps you active. There are lots of different things you can do—exercise isn't just running or aerobic dance or the StairMaster or *any* single activity. In fact, a *combination* of activities—a program of mixing and matching different sports and workout routines, known as cross-training—helps many people stick to their exercise program long after others have grown bored and dropped out.

Sure, if you love your stationary bike or your stepping class or your weekly tennis game, keep it up as long as you're enjoying it. But remember that there are lots of options. The minute you feel a sense of boredom about your workout program, think about switching sports or adding to your repertoire. That change of pace can give you a whole new appreciation for your exercise time.

If you're just starting to become a regular exerciser and are perplexed about which sport(s) to choose, you can't go wrong by beginning with a simple walking program. It's the most popular fitness activity by far, and for good reason: It can be done safely by nearly everyone; you can do it just about anywhere, anytime, alone or with a friend, with or without musical accompaniment; it's simple to adjust the pace and frequency as you do it more and more; and it just makes you feel good to do it—there are few things that beat a brisk walk on a lovely day, whether you're hoofing it through a park, on a country road, in the woods, or on a beach. Regular walking provides many of the health benefits you would derive from any other exercise with far less of the stress and strain on your body and little or no risk of injury. In fact, the exercise program we've outlined below begins with a sport we call PaceWalking, a simple variation on ordinary walking.

Here's Why They Call It "Regular" Exercise

FOR MOST OF US—whether we're large, small, or in between—the difficulty with "regular exercise" is *not* the concept of "exercise" but rather the concept of "regular." If you decide that you want to get exercise into your life, it's a good idea to work on the "regular" part. We suggest, as you'll see below, starting out with ordinary walking, until you've convinced yourself that, yes, you can find or make the time to do this and that you like it. Then, you can go on to choosing one or more sports, if you like, or stick to the walking.

Commitment is the key. A half-hearted, one-shot attempt at exercise—such as vigorously engaging in some sport you've never tried before or haven't done in years—simply won't produce the results you're looking for or make you feel good enough to keep you going. Begin with a few short (10-to-20-minute) workouts. Next, you can decide how many workout sessions you think you can reasonably and realistically fit into your life *on an ongoing basis*—let's say, three times a week. Of course, you can always adjust these numbers up or down as you go. But first you've got to make the commitment to do *something* physical, on a consistent basis. Once you've done your brief workouts, a few times a week for two to four weeks, guess what? You've conquered the problem of "regular exercise"—you've become a regular exerciser!

It's easy to get all fired up about a new program at the beginning, and many of us are. But personal and work obligations, now and in the future, can make it all too easy to go AWOL from your fitness plan. To avoid having that happen to you, you'll see, below, an exercise schedule that can be used for just about any activity you choose, designed to get you going and *keep* you going.

Finding/Making the Time to Exercise

OKAY, WE'RE ALL TOO BUSY to exercise regularly. Now that we've gotten *that* excuse out of the way, here's an interesting little fact you may not know: *Some* of us adults—indeed, between 20 million and 30 million of us—*do* exercise regularly. So, while we can all say we're too busy to exercise, many of us have still decided that it's *worth* carving out the time to make it a permanent part of our lives.

The question is, When will *you* exercise?

As with your choice of *what* activity(ies) you will do and how much you will do them, the matter of *when* you work out is also your choice. Naturally, you'll need to examine your present schedule to see what makes sense for you. If you're like most people, you probably have more free time on the weekends, so you might want to center the majority of your fitness activities around Saturdays and Sundays. (But keep in mind that exercising *only* on the weekend isn't good for your muscles, bones, and joints—you need to work them out at least one day during the week too.) If you work nine to five (give or take) five days a week, your best weekday exercise time may be before or after work. If you're self-employed and/or on the road a lot, your workout-time options may be more flexible. If you exercise with a spouse or a friend, your exercise schedule will be determined at least in part by that of your workout partner.

If any generality about scheduling exercise can be made, it's that many people find that exercising early in the day—before things get too hectic and too many other obligations start to crowd their calendar—keeps them more faithful to their workout program. What's more, morning exercise provides a psychological lift that lasts all day and helps keep you focused on *all* your health-promoting goals, including healthier eating and stress management. But if you're one of those who like it better before or even after dinner, that's fine too. The best schedule is the one that works for you.

Preventing Exercise Injuries and Health Problems

THE QUICKEST WAY TO SCUTTLE your exercise program—not to mention many of your normal daily activities—is to get injured. Here's how to make sure that doesn't happen to you:

• Let your health-care professional know you plan to begin a regular exercise program, as well as what kind of exercise you intend to do, and get an okay. This is particularly critical if you have been diagnosed with any chronic health problem, such as coronary artery disease (signified by, for example, a heart attack or angina) or lung disease, or have a history of heart-related illness. Also, if you have any type of weight-related problem, such as osteoarthritis in your knees, your doctor may suggest that you limit the type and intensity of your workout.

• Ease into it. You don't want to take the chance of overtaxing your heart, especially if you're over 40 and fairly sedentary. So take it easy, particularly at the beginning.

• If you're doing any kind of exercise other than simple walking (where injury is pretty uncommon), it's a good idea to do 5 to 10 minutes of warming up, followed by some easy stretches, before you start your workout. Why are warming up and stretching so important? The warm-up increases blood circulation to the muscles, and the stretching further prepares them for the more strenuous activity to follow. You can warm up with just 2 or 3 minutes of marching in place, riding a stationary bike at a moderate pace, or calisthenics. When you stretch, do it slowly, holding a muscle in a stretched-out position for 10 to 30 seconds. After your workout, give your body a chance to recover slowly by cooling down: simply continue the activity you were doing, but at a slower pace, for 2 or 3 minutes. (For more information on stretching, we recommend *Great Shape: The First Fitness Guide for Large Women* by Pat Lyons and Debby Burgard [Bull Publishing Company] for its clear photographs and sensitivity to large-size people.)

• When exercising, *stop* the minute you feel any pain or tightness in your chest or *any* pain in your body that doesn't feel simply like soreness in previously unused muscles or the brief ache that accompanies pushing your muscles really hard. (Sudden, sharp pain is usually a sign that something not quite right has happened.) Also, slow down or stop completely as soon as you feel you're doing too much. Pushing yourself beyond your physical limit makes you highly susceptible to injury.

• Wear the right shoes for the exercise you're doing. If you're a beginner, go to a sporting-goods shop or athletic-footwear store and get the advice of an *experienced* salesperson to make sure you're buying the right kind of shoe for the exercise you intend to do. Also, periodically check the soles of your shoes to make sure they're not worn down. Once you become a regular exerciser and you're doing a sport like walking or running, don't be surprised if your shoes need replacing as often as every three months or so.

• Drink plenty of water or other noncaloric fluid throughout the day. This is always a good idea but particularly when you're exercising and depleting your body's water supply. Get your fill of fluids *before* you feel thirsty so you don't risk dehydration, especially if you're exercising in warm weather.

• And speaking of the weather, be sure to take it into account when you head outdoors to do your workout. You can exercise in cold temperatures if you wish, as long as you dress in layers of clothing that "breathe" as your body warms up and you begin to sweat. When the outdoor temperatures climb, you may be more comfortable doing your walking at an air-conditioned mall or on the local high school walking track.

Setting Your Exercise Goals

IN CHAPTER FOUR, WE DISCUSSED how important it is for you to set health-promotion goals—essential to getting and staying focused—and to be realistic about what you can do while at the same time exploring your limits. Goal-setting is especially important when it comes to exercise. Indeed, the exercise goals you set may well be the most critical ones of all your health-promotion goals. Why? Because, as we said earlier, setting the goal of "becoming a regular exerciser" means that you've made the commitment to yourself to make exercise an ongoing part of your life, putting in some time doing it every week (if not every day).

If you've decided you are going to engage in regular exercise, your first goal should be to establish in your own mind why you're doing this and what you want to accomplish. Do you want to minimize the health-risk factors associated with a sedentary lifestyle? Do you want to feel more energetic or feel better about yourself? Do you want to increase your strength and physical fitness?

As an overweight person who may have had a lot of trouble losing weight in the past, you should make it clear to yourself that this time you're going to be exercising for the sake of the *exercise* and for such benefits as enhancing your enjoyment of life, giving you more energy, and perhaps toning your muscles. It's critical that you don't create a hidden agenda for yourself—that is, exercising in the hope of losing weight. Because, as you know, that will not necessarily be the result. If that's something you're secretly hoping for or expecting, you may end up feeling very frustrated and lose any pleasure and benefits you can derive from regular exercise.

Therefore, if you still have not yet come to terms with your present weight—accepting the idea that this may be, more or less, what you will weigh for the rest of your life—then this is an excellent opportunity to do so, just before you launch your exercise program. Yes, it's true that exercise *will* help some people take off pounds, and wouldn't it be terrific if you were one of them—but you may not be. So as an overweight person setting your exercise goals, keep your focus on the outcomes other than weight loss.

Initially, as we've noted, your exercise goal should be to make exercise a *habit*. Now's when you need to remind yourself that, whatever your other obligations may be, this special time you've set aside for exercise is yours and yours alone. Once you begin to follow your exercise schedule—whether it's first thing in the morning, after the kids have gone off to school, during a lunch break at work, or before or after dinner—you'll discover that you've begun to *feel* better. You may not see any changes in your body but if you're like most people, you'll definitely notice a change in your attitude. What's happening? For one thing, you've begun to take control, to take greater responsibility for yourself. You've deliberately added a new, ongoing activity to your day-to-day life, something that in itself can make you feel more vigorous and healthy throughout the day. It's a wonderful feeling—so wonderful, in fact, that you'll soon stop worrying about what the exercise is (or isn't) doing to your weight and simply start enjoying it for its own sake.

It's very likely that your weekly or monthly exercise goals will change over time. That's because 1) your level of fitness will increase and you may want to continue to challenge your body's abilities and 2) you'll probably want to add variety to your exercise routine by periodically switching activities, which may mean setting different goals for the particular activity you choose. The exercise program we've outlined below will help you progress gradually from one stage to the next.

An Exercise Program for Life

As we said earlier, walking is the best and simplest exercise for most people, regardless of your initial fitness level. But the five tables that follow (starting on page 143), each covering 13 weeks, can be used with *any* sport or fitness activity you prefer. They start with an Introductory Program all the way up through what we call a Maintenance Double-Plus Program, and you will see that they take you from an easy 30 minutes a week all the way up to an average (over 13 weeks) of 240 minutes (or four hours) a week for ambitious exercisers.

You'll see that all of these workout programs are measured in minutes, not miles. That makes them interchangeable for any of the sports you might wish to do. In addition, you will derive far greater benefit from your workout if you focus on the *time* you spend working out, not on the particular number of steps, blocks, or miles you cover or the speed at which you move. Why? A time goal is much easier to achieve and maintain than a speed or distance goal. Psychologically, it's much easier to walk for 40 minutes, say, than to try to cover three or four miles at a particular clip.

What's more, you can easily vary your speed and distance, depending on how you feel and what the conditions are like. On days when you're full of energy and the weather's nice, chances are you'll just naturally *want* to walk faster and longer. Then, within the time allotted for that day's workout, you'll be going a greater distance. But there will be no pressure to do so—going more slowly and for less time on a given day will be fine too. So regardless of the sport or activity you choose, *minutes* spent exercising should be the common denominator. Work out at your own pace, but try to work out for the full amount of time you've set aside for it.

Take a look at Tables 6-1 through 6-5. They present easy, 13-week sets of workouts that have been designed for a regular exerciser—or for those of you who expect to become one soon.

If you look at Table 6-1, you'll see that it starts with ordinary walking for 30 minutes a week, 10 minutes per day, three times a week, just to get you going and focused on the "regular" aspect of exercise. By the end of the first 13-week Introductory block, it has you doing what we call PaceWalking for a full 90 minutes a week. (See the mini glossary, page 149, for a definition of PaceWalking.) But to get there, you will have averaged only one hour per week for the 13 weeks.

The Developmental Program in the next 13 weeks (Table 6-2) takes you up to 180 minutes (three hours) a week by the end, but this time, you will be averaging two hours a week over the 13 weeks. While that might seem a bit intimidating at first, remember that it comes a full *26 weeks* into the program. You will have built, slowly and gradually over a half-year period, from 30 minutes to 180 minutes per week, so it's quite likely your body will be ready and even eager for that additional activity.

We have then provided you with *three* Maintenance Programs (Tables 6-3, 6-4, and 6-5). Why so many? Because we want you to have choices. The maintenance phase provides you with an average of two hours a week of exercise over 13 weeks. That's plenty to get most of the benefits of regular exercise. But then there's Maintenance Plus, for an average of three hours per week over 13 weeks, and Maintenance Double-Plus, averaging four hours a week. Many regular exercisers do average three to four hours per week on an ongoing basis. Thus, these three different maintenance programs give you the opportunity (if you want it) to challenge your body's capabilities over time.

We're assuming that, after you've been a regular exerciser for a half-year, it's going to be such an important part of your life that you might want to push your personal envelope and see how far you can comfortably go. But keep in mind that you can also choose to level off at *any* maintenance phase. If, for example, you prefer to keep your workouts along the lines of Table 6-3, rather than Table 6-4 or 6-5, that's fine. As we've said before, the "exercise" component of regular exercise is critical, but so is the "regular," and whatever helps you the most in keeping it up is what we recommend.

You'll notice that in the programs presented in Tables 6-2, 6-4, and 6-5, more than half the total workout time is scheduled for the weekends, so that doing it becomes more convenient for most folks. In addition, you have several days off during each week. Plus, there's a full week off at the beginning of each new stage of the program in order to give your body a chance to regroup and get ready for the next level of exercise.

Following this three-stage program—Introductory, Developmental, and Maintenance, at whichever level is comfortable for you—will allow you, regardless of your size, current fitness level, or exercise history, the chance to become a regular exerciser in the simplest way possible: slowly, gradually, and without the need to make an overwhelming time commitment.

Table 6-1: The Just the Weigh You Are Exercise Plan

PHASE I
INTRODUCTORY PROGRAM
(TIMES IN MINUTES)

Week	M	T	W	Th	F	S	S	Total	Comments
1	Off	10	Off	10	Off	Off	10	30	Ordinary walking
2	Off	10	Off	10	Off	Off	10	30	Ordinary walking
3	Off	20	Off	20	Off	Off	20	60	Ordinary walking
4	Off	20	Off	20	Off	Off	20	60	Ordinary walking
5	Off	20	Off	20	Off	Off	20	60	Fast walking
6	Off	20	Off	20	Off	Off	20	60	Fast walking
7	Off	20	Off	20	Off	Off	30	70	Fast walking
8	Off	20	Off	20	Off	Off	30	70	Fast walking
9	Off	20	Off	20	Off	Off	20	60	PaceWalking
10	Off	20	Off	20	Off	Off	30	70	PaceWalking
11	Off	20	Off	30	Off	Off	30	80	PaceWalking
12	Off	20	Off	30	Off	Off	30	80	PaceWalking
13	Off	30	Off	30	Off	Off	30	90	PaceWalking

Table 6-2: The Just the Weigh You Are Exercise Plan

PHASE II
DEVELOPMENTAL PROGRAM
(TIMES IN MINUTES)

WEEK	M	T	W	TH	F	S	S	TOTAL
1	Off	Off	Off	Off	Off	Off	Off	Off
2	Off	20	Off	20	Off	Off	20	60
3	Off	20	Off	20	Off	20	20	80
4	Off	20	Off	20	Off	20	30	90
5	Off	20	Off	30	Off	20	30	100
6	Off	20	Off	30	Off	20	40	110
7	Off	30	Off	30	Off	30	30	120
8	Off	30	Off	30	Off	30	40	130
9	Off	30	Off	40	Off	30	40	140
10	Off	30	Off	40	Off	30	50	150
11	Off	40	Off	30	Off	30	60	160
12	Off	40	Off	30	Off	40	60	170
13	Off	30	Off	40	Off	50	60	180

Table 6-3: The Just the Weigh You Are Exercise Plan

PHASE III
MAINTENANCE PROGRAM
(TIMES IN MINUTES)

WEEK	M	T	W	TH	F	S	S	TOTAL
1	Off	Off	Off	Off	Off	Off	Off	Off
2	Off	30	Off	30	Off	40	Off	100
3	30	Off	40	Off	20	Off	40	130
4	Off	40	Off	30	Off	40	Off	110
5	30	Off	40	Off	20	Off	40	130
6	Off	40	Off	30	Off	60	Off	130
7	20	Off	30	Off	30	Off	40	120
8	Off	40	Off	30	Off	50	Off	120
9	20	Off	40	Off	20	Off	60	140
10	Off	30	Off	30	Off	40	Off	100
11	20	Off	30	Off	20	Off	40	110
12	Off	40	Off	30	Off	60	Off	130
13	20	Off	30	Off	30	Off	40	120

Table 6-4 : The Just the Weigh You Are Exercise Plan

PHASE III
MAINTENANCE PLUS PROGRAM
(TIMES IN MINUTES)

	M	T	W	TH	F	S	S	TOTAL
WEEK								
1	Off	Off	Off	Off	Off	Off	Off	Off
2	Off	30	Off	40	Off	30	50	150
3	Off	30	Off	50	Off	40	60	180
4	Off	40	Off	40	Off	50	80	210
5	Off	30	Off	50	Off	40	60	180
6	Off	50	Off	30	Off	50	70	200
7	Off	40	Off	30	Off	30	60	160
8	Off	30	Off	50	Off	40	60	180
9	Off	30	Off	40	Off	30	50	150
10	Off	30	Off	50	Off	40	50	170
11	Off	40	Off	30	Off	50	70	190
12	Off	40	Off	40	Off	50	80	210
13	Off	30	Off	50	Off	40	60	180

Table 6-5: The Just the Weigh You Are Exercise Plan

PHASE III
MAINTENANCE DOUBLE-PLUS PROGRAM
(TIMES IN MINUTES)

WEEK	M	T	W	TH	F	S	S	TOTAL
1	Off	Off	Off	Off	Off	Off	Off	Off
2	Off	30	40	Off	30	40	70	210
3	Off	30	50	Off	40	50	70	240
4	Off	40	40	Off	50	60	80	270
5	Off	30	50	Off	30	50	80	240
6	Off	50	30	Off	30	60	90	260
7	Off	40	30	Off	30	50	70	220
8	Off	30	50	Off	30	60	70	240
9	Off	30	40	Off	30	50	60	210
10	Off	30	50	Off	30	60	70	240
11	Off	40	30	Off	40	60	80	250
12	Off	40	40	Off	40	60	90	270
13	Off	30	50	Off	30	70	60	240

Exercise Glossary

Quite a few key words and phrases are used to describe various aspects of regular exercise. In case you're not familiar with all of them, this mini glossary should help:

aerobic exercise: literally, exercising "with oxygen." Exercise using large muscle groups (such as the arms and shoulders or buttocks and legs) that is intense enough to cause a significant increase in muscle oxygen uptake. Aerobic exercise includes such activities as jogging and swimming. If, during exercise, your pulse reaches or exceeds 60 percent of your maximum normal age-adjusted heart rate (see *maximum heart rate*, below), you are considered to be exercising aerobically. An even simpler way of determining whether you are exercising aerobically: You have probably reached an aerobic level if you are breathing hard and sweating in mild-to-cold outdoor temperatures.

anaerobic exercise: literally, exercising "without oxygen." Intense physical activity, of necessity very short in duration, fueled by energy sources within the contracting muscles without the use of inhaled oxygen. Weight training is an anaerobic exercise.

"burn": the feeling of heat or intense pain of short duration in a muscle or group of muscles when you are exercising that part of your body. You know you've succeeded in isolating a muscle group when you feel the burning sensation there, which indicates that the area isn't getting enough oxygen. This is a normal part of anaerobic activity.

maximum heart rate: theoretically, the maximum rate at which your heart can beat per minute at your age. The general formula for your maximum heart rate is 220 minus your age. If you're a beginner, you should not exceed 65 percent of your maximum normal age-adjusted heart rate. After the first 13 weeks or so, you can start working up toward a maximum of 80 percent, if desired.

nonaerobic exercise: any physical activity above the normal resting state involving one or more major muscle groups that is sustained but not so intense as to cause a significant increase in muscle oxygen uptake, such as strolling.

PaceWalking (also known as health walking or power walking): an aerobic exercise done as follows: You walk fast, with a purposeful stride of medium length. With each step, land on your heel, then roll forward along the outside of the foot, and push off with your toes. Try to keep your feet pointed straight ahead, walking on an imaginary line, which will help your balance and rhythm and allow you to increase your speed, if you wish. Keep your back straight but not rigid, your shoulders dropped and relaxed, and your head up. Swing your arms strongly as you walk, with elbows comfortably bent.

recovery heart rate: your heart rate measured at the end of your workout after cooling down. It is used to determine when the heart rate has returned to its normal, pre-exercise pulse.

weight training (also known as strength training or resistance training): the process of increasing muscle strength (the ability to lift heavy objects) and muscular endurance (the ability to repeat a movement requiring strength). It involves repetitive sets of exercises aimed at strengthening specific parts of the body.

A Few More Tips for Following the Exercise Program

• **Don't go to Step 2 until you've mastered Step 1.** If, say, you get to the end of the first four weeks of your exercise program and have trouble—you're huffing and puffing throughout your workout, for example—do *not* be a martyr and go on to Week 5. Instead, go back to Week 1 or 2 and take it nice and slow, completing your workout without straining. Remember, your goal is to become a regular exerciser. If all goes well, you'll be doing this for the rest of your life, so if it takes an extra four, six, or eight weeks at the beginning to master your program, it's worth it.

• **Intensity is important—up to a point.** Don't get too hung up about how intense your workout needs to be; it's really up to you. Studies have shown that virtually *any* regular exercise that we do is beneficial, so even if your intensity level is fairly low, whatever you're doing is still better than nothing. However, chances are you will eventually be reaching a level of intensity that's at least at the lower end of the aerobic range—which means you will be doing your cardiovascular system and other body systems a lot of good. Activities that can produce a moderate level of intensity (expending between four and seven calories per minute) include brisk walking (at 3 to 4 mph), bicycling (up to 10 mph), and swimming with moderate effort.

Gradual Change Leads to Permanent Changes

SLOW AND STEADY SHOULD BE YOUR MOTTO, particularly if your backside tends to spend more time in a Barcalounger than on a bicycle seat. Don't try to do too much all at once. For now, a reasonable and manageable goal would be, just as is laid out in Table 6-2, "I will walk for 10 minutes, at a normal pace, three times a week." Then, after doing this for two weeks, you increase the length of each walk by 10 minutes for the next two weeks, and so on throughout the program. If you want to add an extra session now and then, that's fine, but you don't have to. After you have been walking for a few weeks, you will probably find yourself picking up speed, but you don't have to do that either.

Again, what's crucial is to create an exercise program that's reasonable for *you,* one you feel is comfortable and fun. You're not in training to run a 10K road race or a marathon. (Although, who knows? Someday doing a race might become a goal for you.) And certainly, if you're already fairly fit and want to move more quickly through the program we outlined above, you have our blessing. Just don't attempt too much too soon, which can lead to pain, possible injury, and an increased likelihood of quitting.

For now, your aim is to *begin* to exercise, *continue* to exercise, and *maintain* a schedule and pace that are challenging without being overwhelming. Success leads to further success. Give yourself the opportunity to taste the success that comes with being a regular exerciser. Do that, and you're bound to want to keep it up. A *gradual* increase in time spent and, if you're so motivated, in speed and distance covered are the ingredients for an exercise program you can live with for life.

Making Exercise a Part of Your Daily Life

DEPENDING ON HOW COMMITTED you are to upping your fitness level and how much time you feel you can spend, exercise can be anything from an hour of vigorous aerobic exercise all the way down to simply increasing your current level of daily activity by about 30 minutes several times a week. For those of us who do most of our workouts in the form of housework, "exercise" has been officially expanded to include such common day-to-day activities as mowing the lawn (yes, even with a power mower!), home repairs, and housecleaning. Even if you don't want to PaceWalk, swim, or play volleyball, you'll be doing your heart and your overall health a world of good if you simply try to rack up an accumulated 30 minutes a day of the kinds of activities listed below:

Activity	Calories burned per hour for a 175-pound woman
Gardening (digging)	375
Gardening (hoeing)	504
Grocery shopping	200
Housecleaning	252
Mopping the floor	267
Raking leaves	236
Scrubbing the floor	456
Shoveling snow	614
Vacuuming	200
Washing the car	236
Window washing	252

Here are a few more suggestions for working exercise into your usual routine:

• Use the stairs instead of the elevator. (If you work or live on the 39th floor, walk partway.)

• Get off the subway one stop from your destination (or get off the bus a couple of stops) and walk the rest of the way.

• If you live within a mile or two of work or school, walk or bike there in good weather instead of driving or using public transportation.

• When you drive, park at the far end of the lot or even at *another* lot a half-mile or so from your destination and walk the rest of the way.

• Walk to the supermarket and bring home your groceries the old-fashioned way: in a shopping cart or wagon.

• Walk to the mall. If it's too far away, park your car in the mall lot as far away from the buildings as possible.

Tips from a Trainer

Caroline Rubin is a Philadelphia-area certified aerobics instructor who, among other things, teaches fitness classes for large-size people. Here are some of the words of wisdom she shares with her clients:

- **Exercising is not a contest.** Don't do something just because everyone else is doing it. Not all knee lifts have to reach your chest. If you learn to listen to your body, it will tell you everything you need to know.

- **Fitness levels vary.** When you begin, your fitness level may be quite low. But don't give up! The object is to get to a state where you are physically (cardiovascularly) fit, even if you are overweight. There is no magic formula to get to an advanced state of fitness—it takes perseverance. And it's worth it!

- **Each time you work out, push yourself a little.** This way, you are always advancing to the next fitness level.

- **Slowly start doing some weight-bearing exercises.** Weight-bearing exercises improve your bone density (making you less prone to developing osteoporosis), increase your lean muscle mass, and cause you to burn more calories when you exercise. Buy a set of 2-pound and 5-pound weights for this purpose. Get a book on weight lifting, or read one of the many exercise magazines that cover this subject. Incorporate *slow, gentle* weight-lifting exercises into your routine every other day if you can.

- **Remember, you aren't merely exercising—you are mapping out a new lifestyle for yourself.** This takes time, so be patient but tenacious! You will want to quit at times. But if you persevere, you will begin to feel so good—and feel so good about yourself—that you will want to keep going.

Staying Motivated for Life/ Making Exercise Fun

THE KEY TO REMAINING A REGULAR EXERCISER is in keeping your exercise motivation mobilized, which we discussed in Chapter Four. One way to keep going is by periodically reviewing your fitness goals, remembering just *why* you're waking up an extra hour earlier three days a week so you can get in your Pace-Walking or that racquetball game. This will help you stay focused on the value of your workouts.

Then there's that old motivational trick we call *making it fun.* Even if you've always hated exercise or couldn't sustain a workout program for any length of time, our theory is that you simply never found the right activity or learned how to make it fun for *you.* Below are some ways to add some zip to your workouts:

- Listen to books on tape or your favorite CDs while walking.
- Reserve your at-home workout time to catch up with your favorite magazines or television news shows while you're walking on the treadmill, or talk to a friend on a portable phone while riding your exercise bike.
- Buy yourself a new exercise outfit that makes you feel good.
- Get a dog and go for regular walks or runs with your pet.
- End your workout with a pleasant ritual you can look forward to. How about a soak in a scented bathtub (instead of a hurried shower)? A tall glass of your favorite cool beverage while relaxing in your most comfortable chair? A half-hour to do exactly what you want to do?
- Throw a certain amount of money (say, 50 cents or a dollar) into a jar or piggy bank every time you complete a workout session. At the end of a month or two, using the money you've accumulated, splurge on something you want. (The more frivolous, the better.)
- Keep a written record of your exercise progress. Seeing just how far you've come is a terrific motivator and will help keep you interested in your program.

• Enjoy dancing? Remember that any kind of fast dancing is exercise. So look for dance classes in your neighborhood where you can brush up your two-step or your Twist *and* get fit at the same time.

• If you're a walker, jogger, or biker, change your route periodically. Taking a variety of paths will help you maintain your interest—plus, you'll get to know your neighborhood better.

• Think about a nonfitness activity you enjoy, then figure out how to build some exercise into it. For example, if you love to shop, forget the home-shopping channels and let your legs do the walking through the malls or the stores downtown. Like traveling? Make your next vacation a bike tour or week at a ski resort.

• Invite friends for a "fitness date" instead of the usual dinner or drinks. Go walking or hiking through the woods together some Saturday afternoon, or throw a casual party that includes badminton or touch football.

And If You Still Hate to Exercise?

OUR LENGTHY PEP TALK about the value of exercise notwithstanding, it's quite possible that you remain one of those holdouts, someone who still dislikes the mere thought of exercise. What do you do?

Don't do it.

That's right; you heard us. We believe that those folks who truly can't stand to exercise are opening themselves up for problems if they force themselves to do it. Instead of being a benefit, it can turn into a major downer. Too many things can go wrong. For example, if forcing yourself to do this dreaded activity makes you angry, you may actually be more vulnerable to injury. If you're exercising against your will, it won't make you feel energetic, revved up, and positive but rather all the opposite feelings—tired, frustrated, and negative. So if that's the case, what's the point?

But before we end here, we just want to make a couple of other suggestions to you exercise-resisters out there. First, make sure you've given your exercise program a fair shake before you blow it off. The truth is, most people *don't* enjoy exercise immediately; it takes time before the average person can feel and see the benefits. So if you haven't tried it for, say, at least a full month, you're probably being too hasty if you quit now.

This is particularly true if you're trying a new sport that requires practice to perfect (which, frankly, describes just about any sport there is). Okay, so you can't hit a tennis ball very well—but how long have you been trying? Maybe not long enough. (And that's true whether or not you consider yourself to be naturally athletic.) If you're just *starting* to get the hang of rollerblading or jazz-dancing, keep going! Give yourself a chance to get good at it and to like it. Also, remember that while walking, running, or cycling can be boring at times, at the levels we do them, they are no-skill sports.

On the other hand, discovering after some period of time that you happen to be quite adept at lifting a lot of weight, for example, or at putting that ball in just the right place with your racquet, or at running for quite a distance (even if you're not terribly fast) can be a powerful motivator. However, if you truly believe you've given the activity a fair chance and you still feel it's not for you, give yourself permission *not* to do it.

Another thing: Just because you may hate exercise now, it doesn't mean you'll hate it in six months. It may be something as simple as a change in the weather (from winter to spring) or in your schedule (from frantic to fine) or in your state of mind (from stressed-out to calm). So don't feel compelled to launch a full-scale exercise program now if you don't honestly feel you can maintain it. Wait awhile. You may want to give it a whirl later on.

PROFILE

Ellie Hodder

Portland, Oregon
Age: 46
Height: 5'4"
Weight: 220 pounds
Occupation: Certified fitness instructor

LIKE MOST WOMEN MY AGE, I always thought of myself as fat, although it's more likely that I was underfit than overweight. When I opened my coed fitness facility, Corner on Health, in 1988, I weighed about 145 pounds. I got a shock a year later when, due to a medical situation, I gained about 80 pounds, even though I ate carefully and constantly worked out. Believe me, I don't sit at a desk all day eating candy bars. I teach nutrition, and I'm very active.

But suddenly, I had a problem, or so I thought: Here I was, the owner of a relatively new gym. Could I continue to teach health and fitness given my new size? Would I have any credibility with my students? It's what any person would be thinking as she approached 200 pounds. My body just didn't conform to what a body should do if a person were eating right and exercising.

Instead of worrying about it, though, I decided to keep the doors of my gym open and see what happened. I continued doing what I had always done—teaching nutrition and leading exercise classes—and you know what? No one ever said to me, "My workout would be better if *you* were skinnier!" Most people who come to my gym—and stay—are relieved not to have to model themselves after the typical aerobics instructor. Seeing an instructor with a body like theirs who is active, eats well,

PROFILE

and is proactive about her health gives them permission to feel okay about themselves. I know from personal experience that people don't care about the size of the instructor—they just want honesty and real information from that person.

I would say there's probably a good chance that my weight has something to do with hormones—when certain hormones are out of balance, my weight will definitely go up. I can drop a few pounds by cutting calories, but it takes extreme measures, and I also know that it's not something all large women can do. While it might be better for me to lose some weight, there is still a lot of documentation proving that large, active people are at lower health risk than people who are skinny and inactive, so I refuse to worry about it. I teach 8 to 10 aerobics classes a week, and I walk 20 to 40 miles a week. Physically, I can do what I want most of the time. I have asthma, but exercise helps me manage the symptoms more easily—there's a well-documented link between exercise and the management of lung disease. I began exercising before I knew I had asthma, and I certainly wouldn't stop exercising, even with asthma. I *love* to exercise.

I wish my husband exercised more, and I tease him about it sometimes, but fortunately we have two dogs, and he and I take them for long walks. Since meeting my husband, I gained 30 pounds, but it hasn't hurt our marriage—my husband loves me, period, and I love him, period. If you're in a loving relationship and you believe your partner is compromising her safety or health, of course you'll want to say something, but that's not necessary here. Unfortunately, not all mates are as understanding as mine is.

The myth of weight creates many victims; some people will do almost anything to try to lose weight. Lots and lots of people come to my classes [to try to get back on track] after excessive dieting. I have one woman who trained for a marathon

PROFILE

by putting herself on a fasting program; she lived on protein drinks. Two and a half years later, she's still struggling to maintain her weight on 1,700 calories a day. Dieting screws up the body terribly.

Even with all our sophisticated testing and research, medical science doesn't truly understand the causes of weight gain. There can be many reasons for it. For example, certain medications can cause hunger signals and weight gain. The medical and weight-loss communities are not honest with people, nor are they very successful—you'd never go to a doctor with the track record of a typical person in the diet industry.

But these people aren't the only ones at fault. We Americans have a responsibility to get our butts out the door, exercise on a regular basis, and eat better food. I saw one study recently that said only 18 percent of Americans exercised in the last two weeks. There isn't nearly enough emphasis on the connection between physical activity and health. People continue to believe two prevalent myths about weight: one, that if you're fat, it's your fault, and two, that everything can be solved by cutting calories. Neither is true—if they were, we'd be a slim society rather than one becoming increasingly fat. The sad truth is, we're not willing to be proactive about our own lives. I get so sick of hearing, "Yes, but . . ." You can point a finger if you want to, but there's much more that we should and can be doing for ourselves. Being fat may not be my preference, but as a result of my weight, I've gained an understanding of who and what I am. A lot of things could have happened in my life—I could have developed diabetes, I could have had a limb amputated. In the scheme of things, being fat isn't so bad. I have a happy marriage and wonderful friends. I'm grateful that I can do so many, many things. There are so many worse things that can befall a person than being fat.

PROFILE

Carnie Wilson

Los Angeles, California
Age: 28
Height: 5'4"
Weight: "Nicely over 200 pounds"
Occupation: Singer

I STARTED GAINING WEIGHT at age 4. I lived in a real crazy household with my father [Beach Boys singer/songwriter] Brian Wilson [who had problems with drugs and obesity], and that was a scary thing. So I turned to food.

Unfortunately, as I got older, I kept those early eating habits. I've been heavy ever since, except for eight years ago, when I lost 96 pounds. I had always told myself, "When I turn 20, I'll lose the weight," and I did. My sister Wendy, Chynna Philips, and I were bringing out our *Wilson Philips* album, and I was nervous about appearing in public as a heavy person. But after we started our promotion tour, which meant traveling to five cities a day, I started eating cheesecake and hot chocolate at three in the morning. Over the next year and a half, the weight slowly came back.

I felt bad, of course, but I think it happened because I was never really comfortable in my new body—I didn't know how to feel about myself. I would look at my stomach and say, "It's flabby." I didn't look the way I expected to look as a thin person. I'm sure it had to do with my self-image—I was probably better looking than I thought I was.

Today, my body feels very familiar to me. Although I might want to take off 50 pounds for health reasons—I'm concerned because diabetes runs in my family—my weight doesn't stop

PROFILE

me from doing what I want to do. I have talent and something to offer the world. I'm planning my next album, and I'm working on a deal for a line of clothing for large-size women. I've always had boyfriends, and now I'm engaged to a wonderful guy. I love people, and I love life. What I've tried to do all my life is to rely on my personality so people wouldn't focus so much on my weight, and it's worked.

Another reason I convey the sense that I'm comfortable with my body is that I care about how I present myself. I'm interested in fashion, and I like to dress well and be attractive. A lot of people who are heavy lose interest in themselves and let themselves go, but not me—I've always gotten facials, pedicures, manicures, body scrubs. I love perfume, and I love to smell feminine—and you definitely don't have to be thin to look or feel feminine. It's hard to *always* love your body, but I say that, even if you're over 200 pounds, you'll feel better about yourself if you pamper your body. I'm a size 22, and sometimes I think, If only I were a size 14, I could shop in the "normal" section of department stores. At the same time, though, I'm totally excited by what I see these days in larger women's sizes—there's so much more available now. If you want to look good, whatever size you are, it's easier than ever.

Idrea Lippman, the fitness instructor who worked with me on my exercise video, *Great Changes*, really inspired me to love my body more. I may make jokes about my body, like, "My inner thighs have been close friends for a long time!" But at the same time, I've learned to appreciate the beauty of being a woman. I feel shapely, and I'm very happy with certain body parts, such as my legs and my butt. What's more, I've always exercised, so I'm firm. I work out twice, sometimes three times, a week. I usually do an aerobic workout for at least 20 to 35 minutes, plus toning, including leg lifts. I walk a lot—my fiancé and I take our dogs for a walk. And I love sports—swim-

PROFILE

ming, volleyball, and roller skating, and my mom is dying for me to start golfing, so that's also a possibility. I believe that exercising my whole life has helped keep my heart strong, and I have no health problems.

My goal right now is not to look like anyone else—it's to be as healthy as I can. That may eventually include losing some weight, and when I'm at the right weight for me, I'll know it. If I sound confident, it's because all my life, I've surrounded myself with very supportive people. They don't push me or put me down; they only encourage me. If the people in your life aren't supportive, don't listen to what they say; you may be fine just as you are. Look in the mirror, and if you're *not* happy with what you see, change it. We're all more powerful than we think.

CHAPTER SEVEN

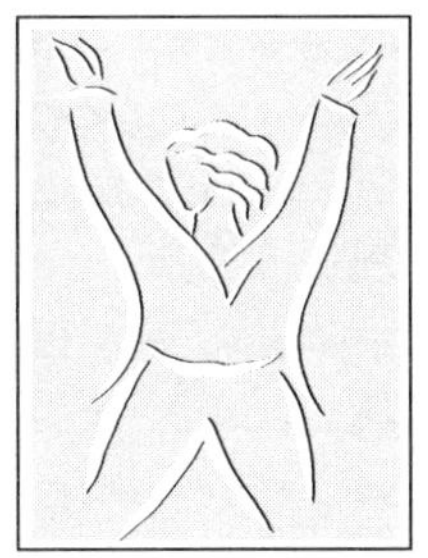

THE BIG PICTURE PLAN *for* HEALTH:

Managing Your Stress and Negative Moods

ARE YOU STRESSED? Join the club! We certainly don't mean to minimize the daily pressures you're under, but let's face it, stress is currently a big problem for *most* people. Look around. Corporations merge, or CEOs order subordinates to go lean and mean, and people lose jobs in the process. Many of us have to work more than one job to make ends meet, which invariably means stress galore and too little time to do everything else we need to do. Even with one job, we are often stressed in our attempts to fit in all of our responsibilities. Kids, divorce, debts, sick or aging parents, our own health concerns—these are all stressors, and sooner or later, one or more of them is bound to affect you.

And why is stress potentially so bad? Because it literally puts *stress*, or strain, on your body. That can cause all sorts of problems, both short- and long-term, including fatigue, anxiety, insomnia, and the gradual wearing down of body systems, which leads to ill health. Learning how to tame those stress factors can contribute enormously to improving the quality of your life. Not only will that skill help you deal with the problems of the moment, but it can also ward off the disease and illness often associated with unmanaged or poorly managed stress.

Happily, there are lots of ways to get your stress under control. In this chapter, we describe techniques that have proved to be tremendously effective. We're not talking about New Age hocus-pocus, either. For many people, the various relaxation therapies you'll see here can be as effective as or more effective than drug therapy in coping with or heading off chronic pain, high blood pressure, asthma, migraine headaches, and mild depression, to name a few. In fact, the government has been so convinced of the effectiveness of these treatments that the National Institutes of Health has created the Office of Alternative Medicine to encourage the use of these treatments as alternatives to conventional drug and surgery-based medicine, where appropriate. Some of the country's first-rate medical schools, including Harvard and Georgetown, have also slowly begun introducing courses in alternative medicine to treat physical problems that are frequently the result of unmanaged stress.

The Food-Stress Connection

IF YOU'RE READING THIS BOOK, it's quite possible that you were conditioned over the years to cope with stressful or emotionally charged situations by turning to an ever-present "friend": food. That pattern may have led, at least in part, to your current weight.

We know how simple it is to rely on food as a crutch when times get tough. After all, compared with a lot of other mood-altering substances you could use, food is relatively inexpensive and readily available. Until and unless a person becomes overweight, there isn't the stigma attached to, say, eating a cream-filled doughnut that there is to smoking a joint or taking a drink of bourbon at 10 in the morning. The worst thing they might say about you is that you're a junk-food junkie—big deal. What's more, it's hard to resist the lift you get (even if it *is* fleeting) from your favorite delicious food.

For many of us, the habit of using food as a tranquilizer or mood elevator started in childhood. Scrape your knee or get taunted in the schoolyard, and there would likely be a loving parent waiting at home, ready to soothe you with a cookie or a dish of rice pudding. (Mom would have done us a lot more good giving us a fat-free hug instead.) Or you may have grown up in a household where it was taught that expressing strong feelings—anger, disappointment, sadness, frustration—was "bad." And so we learned literally to "swallow" our feelings, with the help of food, of course.

As a result, leaning on food for comfort or stress relief may be a very familiar, though possibly damaging, experience. Even if you're now able to accept your weight, you may continue to believe that turning to food in times of trouble or anxiety is okay. After all, you may rationalize, you're no longer trying to lose weight, so what's a few more pounds here and there?

But as we've said earlier in this book, while food should not be looked upon as the enemy, neither should it be relied upon as your pick-me-up buddy when things go wrong. Food, first and foremost, is meant to provide your body with nutrition and energy. Overeating—particularly overeating foods that are high in fat, sugar, and/or sodium—will only set back your present health-promotion program and might, in time, exacerbate any health problems you may now have. Like smoking cigarettes or drinking to excess, eating for stress management doesn't help you get to the heart of the matter and may actually leave you feeling worse about whatever it is that's troubling you or stressing you.

Stress, while unavoidable at times, *can* be handled successfully and foodlessly. Work on mastering one or more of the stress-busting techniques, below. If you do, not only will you be able to handle your immediate source of stress, but you also will have a clearer mind so that you can get your problem in focus—and maybe even come up with a terrific solution.

Assess Your Stress

YOU CAN'T LEARN HOW TO MANAGE your stress until you figure out the *sources* of that stress. First, you should be aware that stress comes in many shapes and sizes (like people!) and that some stress is actually *good*. You can, for example, be stressed as much by the excitement of getting married as by the sadness of getting divorced. Losing a job is one form of stress; so is giving birth to a beautiful, beloved baby.

In general terms, we can define stressors as those demands placed on you by others, by yourself, or by circumstances within or outside your control. Yours might be the chronic stress associated with a frustrating job or an unsatisfying marriage, or it could be sudden and unexpected stress—just as you're starting to make some positive changes in your life and health, something dramatic happens and you're tempted to slip back into some old, bad habit. For example, you might get an injury that discourages you from returning to your exercise program.

How do you keep stress from messing you up? First, you have to analyze the source of your stress. What's stressing you out right now? What tends to stress you out much of the time? Below, check off all the events that currently affect (or recently affected) you:

____**Major life stressors**, such as divorce or marriage/remarriage; death of a spouse, parent, or close friend; death or birth of a child; moving; coping with a chronically ill spouse, parent, or child; your own illness; etc.

____**Money problems:** loss of a job/extended unemployment; mounting bills and not enough money to pay them; investments gone bad; etc.

____**Relationship conflicts**, such as those with a spouse, a child, a boss or co-worker, or a friend.

____**Time shortages** (too much to do and too little time in which to do it).

____**Relatively minor ongoing hassles**, such as crank phone calls, traffic congestion while commuting, noisy neighbors, etc. (Don't underestimate these! They can add up to major stress.)

____**Self-inflicted stress**, such as holding onto anger much longer than is necessary/healthy; being a poor manager of your time, causing unnecessary lateness and delays (different from the time problems described above); habitually finding yourself in bad relationships; etc.

Next, think about the way you respond to the stressors in your life. Which of the following responses are typical for you?

When I feel stressed, I . . .

____tend to use food as a tranquilizer/mood elevator.

____overeat at mealtimes.

____snack between meals a lot.

____neglect to eat a healthy meal or skip meals altogether.

____often reach for foods I know I should try to limit, such as chocolate or other high-fat snacks.

____veg out—watch television, hang around the house, or sleep to excess.

____exercise.

____talk it out with a friend or relative.

____have an alcoholic drink.

____smoke a cigarette.

____bite my nails.

____grind my teeth.

____pull/twist my hair.

____feel physical symptoms, such as aches and pains; digestive problems (heartburn, indigestion, diarrhea, or constipation); break out in hives, acne, or eczema; etc.

____feel anxious/restless.

____feel hopeless/depressed.

____feel frustrated.

____feel irritable/I'm unpleasant to be around.

____have emotional outbursts.
____have trouble sleeping.
____overreact to everyday incidents.
____make many mistakes/have accidents.

Keep a Stress-Awareness Diary

ONCE YOU KNOW what your stress-reaction patterns are, you can start to head off your negative responses before they start. And there's no better way to learn *your* particular stress-and-response patterns than by writing them down. For two weeks, use the chart below to keep track of your stressors and the ways in which you normally deal with them, for better or worse:

	Time	Stressful Event	Response/Reaction
Monday			
Tuesday			
Wednesday			
Thursday			
Friday			
Saturday			
Sunday			

	Time	Stressful Event	Response/Reaction
Monday			
Tuesday			
Wednesday			
Thursday			
Friday			
Saturday			
Sunday			

After you've completed this chart, take a good, hard look at it and see what changes you can begin to make. Let's say, for instance, that an argument with your spouse inevitably leads to frustration for you—and a little visit to the refrigerator; or a tantrum; or a depressing feeling of loss of control.

Instead of succumbing to this typical pattern, there are ways you can deal with the argument and the usual aftermath. How? *Identify* and *adjust.* First, *identify* the source of stress as soon as you can, and then *adjust* your reaction by using one of the stress-busting techniques described below. You will soon learn that while you may not be able to control the *factors* that stress you out, you *can* learn to improve your reaction to them. And you can do this by simply engaging in certain stress-management *behaviors*—thereby avoiding the necessity for analyzing what is stressing you and figuring out how to fix it.

Stress-Management Relaxation Exercises

MUSCLE-RELAXATION EXERCISES help many people manage their stress. Most exercises intended to relieve stress and promote calm have four things in common:

1. being in a quiet environment
2. being in a comfortable position
3. adopting a passive, let-it-happen attitude so you can free your mind of gnawing thoughts and negative emotions
4. continuously repeating a calming word or phrase or paying attention to your breathing so you can get focused

Below are a number of exercises. To see which one works best for *you*, experiment with several. Try to do the same one at least once a day for a full week before deciding that it isn't working and moving on to the next.

Progressive Muscle Relaxation

These exercises involve alternately contracting and relaxing various groups of muscles. Before you begin the actual exercises, follow these suggestions:

- As you relax, try to keep your mind free of thoughts and negative emotions.
- When contracting each muscle group, hold thecontraction/tension for 5 seconds.
- When relaxing each muscle group, relax it for 10 to 30 seconds.
- Make sure you feel the contrast between tension and relaxation before moving on to the next muscle group.
- Repeat the contracting and relaxing of each body part (in the order suggested below) twice. If one part of your body feels especially tight, repeat the exercise up to five more times.
- Don't hold your breath. Remember to *keep breathing* throughout the exercises—breathe in with contraction, breathe out with relaxation.

To Do Progressive Muscle Relaxation:

1. Find a comfortable, quiet place to sit. If you're at home, you might want to put soothing sounds on your CD player—relaxing music, the sounds of waterfalls or ocean waves, etc.

2. Get into a comfortable position and close your eyes.

3. Curl your toes under. Feel the tension in your calves. Hold for 5 seconds, then gradually release to a count of 10. Take a slow, deep breath. Repeat.

4. Curl your toes upward. Feel the tension in the front of your lower legs. Hold for 5 seconds, then gradually release to a count of 10. Take a slow, deep breath. Repeat.

5. Press your knees together as tightly as you can. Hold for 5 seconds, then relax to a count of 10. Repeat.

6. Tighten the muscles of your buttocks and thighs. Hold for 5 seconds, then relax for 10 seconds. Repeat.

7. Tighten your stomach muscles. Hold for 5 seconds, then relax for 10 seconds. Repeat.

8. Arch your back by pressing your shoulders toward each other behind you—your shoulder blades should feel as if they're kissing. Hold the tension for 5 seconds, then relax for 10 seconds. Repeat.

9. Clench both hands into fists. Feel the tension in your fists, hands, and forearms. Hold for 5 seconds, then relax for 10 seconds. Repeat.

10. Bend your elbows upward and make a fist to tense the muscles of your upper arms. Hold for 5 seconds, then relax for 10 seconds. Repeat.

11. Tense a series of facial muscles: Wrinkle your forehead as tightly as you can. Squint your eyes hard. Clench your jaw, biting hard. Press your tongue to the roof of your mouth. Do all of these simultaneously for 5 seconds, then relax for 10 seconds. Repeat.

Deep-Breathing Exercises

1. Find a comfortable, quiet place to sit, with soothing music playing in the background, if you like.

2. Close your eyes.

3. Place one hand on your abdomen and the other on your chest.

4. Inhale slowly and deeply through your nose, with the air moving into your abdomen, so that the hand on your abdomen lifts outward and upward as you inhale. Your chest should move only slightly and only when your abdomen moves.

5. Exhale slowly through your mouth.

6. Take long, deep breaths. Notice the sound of your breathing and/or the feeling of your abdomen rising and falling.

Besides calming you, these exercises can also help you get in touch with your body and all its parts, something you may have been reluctant to do until now because of your weight. But making that physical connection with yourself helps you feel more alive and good about yourself, whatever size you happen to be.

Meditation

Meditation is a method of focusing your attention on the present moment so you can better control your thoughts and reactions and experience the here and now. Researchers have found that by concentrating on one thing and learning to "quiet" your mind and body, you become more aware of what's going on both inside and outside yourself. During this process, your body begins to relax—your heartbeat and breathing rate slow down; the blood levels of a natural chemical called lactate (related to stress and fatigue) fall; and there's an increase in the "alpha activity" in the brain, which is yet another sign of relaxation.

Meditation has been used successfully in the treatment of a wide range of health problems, including high blood pressure, heart disease, stroke, and migraine headache. Many people report that using meditation has helped them reinforce the positive health changes they are trying to make.

The exercise we describe below is based on the Relaxation Response, a technique developed by Dr. Herbert Benson, the author of a book by that name and associate professor of medicine at Harvard Medical School. We suggest you start with sessions of 5 to 15 minutes, eventually working up to 30-minute sessions if you like the results. As with the other exercises we've described, the more you do meditation, the better you'll get at it, and the more useful it will be for you:

1. Sit in a chair in a relaxed position, knees comfortably apart and hands resting on your lap. (You may also sit cross-legged on the floor, if you prefer. Place a cushion under your knees for greater comfort.)

2. Choose a short word, syllable, or phrase to concentrate on—"one" and "om" are popular. Start breathing—breathe relaxation in, and breathe tension out. Say the word you've chosen (aloud or silently to yourself) each time you exhale. (Alternatively, each time you exhale, instead of saying your word, concentrate on your body, such as the sensation of your abdomen as it falls.)

3. Close your eyes. Become aware of your breathing. Keep breathing relaxation in and tension out. Continue to breathe slowly and steadily, saying your word as you exhale.

4. Whenever your mind starts to drift—to past thoughts or future events—gently bring your mind back to your breathing and the word you've chosen. Tell yourself that you can always go back to those thoughts later. (This is essential to the success of the exercise. The object is to clear your mind completely, not simply to make quiet time to think about what's troubling you.)

5. When your session is over, sit quietly for a couple of minutes, without using your chosen word. When you're ready, open your eyes.

Assert Yourself!

So far, we have been talking about inner-directed techniques for managing stress. There are *outer*-directed ones you can engage in as well, although they may require some behavior changes to make them work well for you.

We said earlier that stress often comes in the form of demands made upon you by other people. In your life, that person might be a demanding toddler, a demanding boss, or a sister who "demands" that you finally lose some weight "for the sake of your health."

It isn't always easy to positively handle the pressures put on us by others, especially if we care about them (or if they sign our paychecks). Feelings of guilt if we don't do something we "should" do, feelings of obligation to do something for someone we love, or sometimes just plain exhaustion (it's often easier to give in than to fight) frequently dictate our actions in response to the people in our lives and the demands they place on us.

Large-size people may feel an even greater sense of obligation to meet the demands of others. That's because many overweight people feel a tremendous need to please, to be nice, to smooth things over—in short, to be loved. If you succumb to society's notion that Thin is Better Than Fat, you might have believed for a long time (and may *still* believe) that you're at a disadvantage because of your weight. To compensate, you may feel the urge to try to become the perfect daughter or son, the perfect spouse, the perfect parent, the perfect friend. The stress produced by this drive for perfection and by all this people-pleasing can be overwhelming. The consequences can be more than making yourself vulnerable to health problems—you also risk losing your sense of *yourself,* of who you really are.

This is where assertiveness becomes so crucial. It isn't merely a matter of telling your spouse that he'll have to prepare dinner because you have an important meeting to attend or because you're simply too tired to cook tonight, although those are two examples. A more critical need for assertiveness comes from asserting your right to be who you are, at the size you are, without apology or explanation. The real-life stories scattered throughout this book describe people who practice assertiveness skills, ones that they've been able to use in many areas of their lives. The Resources section of this book (starting on page 242) identifies organizations that can help you develop your assertiveness skills; there are also many good books available on this subject. And we'll be talking more about self-acceptance and assertiveness in Chapter Ten.

Laugh!

PERHAPS THE BEST WAY for you to beat stress and see things in perspective is with the help of humor. When you laugh, it's hard to dwell on what's bothering you. Laughter is a highly effective way to distance yourself from the source of the stress that's currently troubling you, short-circuiting those all-too-common feelings of anxiety, helplessness, hopelessness, or whatever else you may feel when you're not managing stress well.

If laughter has been in short supply in your life lately, make it your responsibility—almost as though it were a doctor's written prescription—to "take" something funny for that stressed-out feeling. What invariably makes *you* laugh? Watching a Woody Allen movie or a Richard Simmons video? Rereading *Catch-22*? Playing with your kids or grandkids? Enjoying reruns of your favorite old sitcoms on one of the cable television stations? Make time for a little levity in your life, and you may find that whatever has been worrying you now worries you less.

Learn Time-Management Skills

ALWAYS LATE? Always frantically looking for paper and pen when you're on the phone? Always forgetting important birthdays and appointments? Always saying yes when you should really be saying no? Always discovering things you've misplaced in odd places, like that bologna sandwich in the dresser drawer?

You've got a problem. Call it lack of organization, lack of time-management skills, call it whatever you want. The point is, this behavior pattern can lead to wasted time, missed opportunities, frustration for the people around you—and lots of stress on *you.* Granted, becoming organized after a lifetime of being disorganized may be even harder for you than losing weight—but it's not impossible once you realize that it's crucial for your health to keep your stresses under control.

Think about the folks you know who *are* organized and seem to manage their lives and time effectively. What do they do that you can learn to do too? Many people, for example, find it helpful to have a number of important time-management tools close at hand: an appointment book (paper or electronic); a functioning watch (don't laugh; many people don't wear one); an address book; a notepad to jot down things to remember or act on later; a cellular phone. But even more vital than simply having these items is *using* them on a regular basis and seeing how much more productive and less stressed they can help you become. Starting on page 242, we also recommend a couple of good books on this subject.

Another aspect of streamlining/de-stressing your life is learning to say no when you're overloaded, a challenge for a lot of us. It's a matter of setting priorities in your life—which may well have changed since you first picked up this book. You may now realize that you've been putting yourself and your health on the back burner for too long, a pattern you may now be ready to alter.

As with doing regular exercise and practicing good nutrition, start out by making small changes first. Say no to requests that are relatively inconsequential before moving on to more critical ones. Slowly and gradually, politely reject those nonessential activities and obligations if you feel they're draining you of time and energy you need for yourself. It might take a while for you and the people in your life to get used to the "new you," evolving from the person who almost never refused any request, favor, or project. But your mental and physical well-being depend on your knowing and respecting your time and physical limits and not pushing yourself beyond what's reasonable for you.

Walk Off That Stress

WELL, YOU KNEW you weren't going to escape this chapter without hearing a pitch for the benefits of exercise to ease stress. And for good reason. When you work out hard, your body starts pumping out those mood-elevating endorphins you may have heard of. Endorphins are morphine-like substances released from the pituitary gland during vigorous exercise. If you're the kind of person who likes to work out stresses with a vigorous activity like running, smashing a ball around in a squash court, or boxing, you're apt to feel much better afterwards. But the nice thing is that even *mild* exercise—probably because of its distracting, brain-and-body-relaxing properties—is also a wonderful way to manage stress and improve your mood.

Here are some ways simple walking can help you beat stress:

• If you're so wound up that you think you want to eat something to "calm" yourself down, walk off your jitters instead. As long as you don't walk over to your local doughnut shop, you'll be getting away from the food, and by the time you return, your hunger pangs may well have dissipated.

• Have a problem to solve? Think it through as you walk. Many times, a change of scenery in combination with moving your body helps clarify a resolution to confusing or problematic situations.

• Are you going someplace where traffic is usually a problem—and your blood pressure usually shoots up? Leave the driving to others. Take public transportation part of the way and walk the rest.

• Your boss (or co-worker) is driving you crazy. You *could* scream—*or* you could say, "Excuse me, I'll be back in 15 minutes." Then go out for a walk. Even if it's just a brisk spin around the parking lot, it'll clear your mind and help ease your temper.

• Have something important to discuss with your mate or your teenager? Take them for a stroll to walk and talk it out. Think about how many serious or heartfelt conversations you've had while in the car, avoiding eye contact. For the same reason, you might be able to speak your mind more easily if you're ambling along, side by side.

• Don't forget that walking on a beautiful day, wearing comfortable clothes and the right kind of shoes, is a very pleasant experience in and of itself. Whatever your mood when you leave the house, that walk will often make you feel happier about yourself and more positive about your life.

The 29 Best Stress Busters

When you're feeling beat,
And you wanna eat,
Who you gonna call?
Stress Busters!

Well, it may not have quite the same zing as the original *Ghostbusters* song, but you get the idea. The next time you feel stress getting the best of you, don't automatically reach for that cold pizza in the fridge—reach for this list of great ideas for taking the edge off your negative emotions. Try a different one each time and see which one works best for you.

1. Put on your favorite CD and dance.
2. Take a yoga class.
3. Call a friend.
4. Read a book or magazine.
5. Take a scented bubble bath.
6. Go to the gym.
7. Write your feelings in a journal.
8. Play with your kids or your dog.
9. Get a massage.
10. Go to a movie.
11. Take a walk through the park.
12. Buy yourself (or pick) some flowers.
13. Have sex.
14. Take a catnap.
15. Write a letter to someone you've lost touch with.
16. Stare at a fish tank for 15 minutes (your own or at an aquarium).
17. Flip through an old photo album.
18. Visit a bookstore.
19. Plan your next vacation.
20. Work on your hobby.
21. Sit silently for 10 minutes.
22. Sit on the front porch or stoop and watch the world go by.
23. Do volunteer work.
24. Drop in on a neighbor.
25. Go to a neighborhood coffee bar and sip an exotic blend while you read the newspaper.
26. Pray.
27. Spend 15 uninterrupted minutes catching up with your spouse or your teenager.
28. Walk around the mall and buy yourself a small present.
29. Stop and think about everything in your life that's wonderful.

PROFILE

Sally Strosahl

Aurora, Illinois
Age: 44
Height: 5'6"
Weight: 260 pounds
Occupation: Psychotherapist/marriage and family therapist

I COME FROM STURDY GERMAN FARM STOCK. Both my parents are large, and I grew up as a large kid. I started dieting when I was 10. Now, looking at pictures of myself at that age, I think I wasn't really that big; my size was probably appropriate given my genetics. But then I started messing with my metabolism by dieting and kept doing it until I finally stopped at age 35.

Since becoming a therapist 18 years ago and working with some compulsive overeaters, I can now look back and say I had a mild case of compulsive overeating—but, ironically, only while dieting! When I wasn't dieting, I was able to regulate my food intake quite nicely. And now that I'm not dieting, I'm not troubled by compulsive eating at all.

I've been up and down the scales several times with the typical diets. I never did anything radical like surgery. Just the usual—a water diet, supervised fasting, Weight Watchers . . . I was successful in the short run, in that I would lose 40 to 60 pounds at a time. But then I would gain it back.

I started realizing that dieting was not a good way to lose weight. One of the ways I came to this conclusion was during my early training in grad school, while working with stress management and studying the relationship between stress and illness. I already had a lot of healthy habits in place for my-

PROFILE

self—I was practicing good eating habits, I was a regular exerciser, I didn't smoke cigarettes, I managed stress well. There were very few activities I couldn't do along with my thinner friends; in fact, I lasted longer than some of them! I was then, as I am today, both fit and fat. Yet I was still feeling like something was wrong with me because of my weight.

Then, during my third pregnancy, a health crisis came upon me: I was diagnosed with cervical cancer. It was a turning point for me. That's when I decided to confront my negativity about my body, start thinking positively about myself—and stop dieting. Cervical cancer is not life-threatening when caught early, but I couldn't be treated for it because of my pregnancy. That situation led me to learn a lot about my cancer and deal with it through guided imagery [where you use your mind to focus on good health and positive feelings] and other noninvasive techniques. Through these techniques, I was able to confront the negative messages I had for years been giving myself about my overweight. I came to believe that the bad things I was saying to myself translated to disease in my body. Even though it took a health crisis to get me to that point, I came to feel very comfortable with myself and with the approach to self I now use, which is nondieting and self-affirming-focused.

It's an approach that has caught on around the country. More and more, the media have moved away from dieting to the nondiet approach. Even Weight Watchers now says its program isn't really a diet! Of course, some people will never give up the struggle for a smaller size. If it works in the long run for them, that's fine. But for the majority, for whom it cannot work, there are organizations like Abundia, of which I'm cofounder, which offers support and information to large-size women. Our message is: You'll probably be big the rest of your life, and that's okay. That isn't something everyone wants to hear, and unfortunately, we don't have something too hopeful

PROFILE

or glamorous to replace the dream of thinness with. Many people don't immediately understand the importance of what we're trying to give them. But once they *do* get it, it *is* glamorous for them. Then they can laugh at all the weight-loss fads. There's a great sense of relief—I hear that from many women. And now I'm even getting some requests for information from men.

Yes, the relief is there, but along with that tremendous relief comes an increase in self-responsibility. As soon as you make the decision not to diet anymore, you then have to start making decisions about what's healthy for you. When I say that I'm going to begin tuning in to my body, that's a lot of responsibility—and I don't always know if I'm right in what I'm doing. So giving up dieting is for those who have made it to that level where they're able to give themselves that freedom tied to responsibility.

That isn't easy for people who feel diet shame—all those years of dieting without permanent weight loss can make them feel like failures. They may not feel that they can trust their own appetite signals, and they may not have a sense of their inner wisdom. They need help to wade through all the prescriptions out there.

But once you start to trust your body, it will, as mine does, tell you what's right for you to eat and what isn't. Watch your fat intake by estimating the fat grams in what you eat and how much fat you use in your cooking. I try to eat a low-fat diet not only because I believe it's better for my body but because I know how it feels after I've eaten fatty things—slow and sluggish. My body doesn't like ice cream anymore, but it *does* love nonfat frozen yogurt. I pretty much eat everything, but in moderation. I don't eat a lot of red meat; I'll get a craving for steak about once a month. I'll have an occasional McDonald's hamburger—but not the Quarter Pounder, again because I

PROFILE

don't like how my body feels afterwards. As a family, we'll do stir-fries with lots of vegetables, rice, and beans.

In terms of exercise, I walk outdoors three to four times a week, and I use my NordicTrack three to four times a week. In the summer, I do a lot of biking, and in the winter, cross-country skiing. I'm out there doing a lot of stuff! Being in nature is one way I get into balance.

My body responds well to my program: I do not have high blood pressure, my blood serum cholesterol is low, my blood sugar is normal. All the other health indicators besides my weight are positive for me. My weight hasn't fluctuated at all. I don't weigh myself (and my doctor doesn't either), but I know I'm about the same weight as before—if anything, my body is tighter because I'm fitter.

I also know I'm lucky I'm not in daily pain. (I have a sister who's 5'6" and 120 pounds and lives on painkillers for her arthritis.) Pain in large-size people is not always about weight. I work with supersize people who are in chronic pain, and their doctors say, "If you lost weight, you wouldn't be in such pain," but that's not necessarily true. I try to suggest other ways to help relieve some of that pain, such as adding some fitness activities to their lives—walking around the block, doing chair aerobics, t'ai chi . . . Just learning to breathe differently can help unblock some of the drain on our energy.

It's vital that we large-size people start defining what success is for *us.* We're so inundated with messages that say we can't feel good about ourselves unless we're losing weight, and we tell ourselves, "I'm eating sensibly, I'm exercising—I should be losing weight! What am I doing wrong?" The answer for many large-size people is: Nothing. If success is—as I believe it is—being as healthy as I am in the body I am in now, then what does it matter what the scale says?

PROFILE

Aleta Walker

Castro Valley, California
Age: 39
Height: 5'7"
Weight: 345 pounds
Occupation: Hospital management

I'VE BEEN FAT ALL MY LIFE. I first started dieting when I was about 12 years old. I think I've been on every diet and I've done everything possible to lose weight, with the exception of weight-loss surgery, which I once seriously considered. All that was before I learned to accept myself the way I am.

It's been on ongoing process, but I don't think you can live in a looks-oriented society like ours and accept yourself as a fat person overnight. About 10 years ago, I went into therapy. I had a wonderful therapist who worked with me using visualization exercises. At the time I started therapy, there was only one part of my body that I liked: my ankles. I believed the rest of me was awful because I was so fat. So my therapist and I started by appreciating my ankles—admiring them in the mirror, taking pictures of them. Then, we would take another body part that wasn't so bad. Eventually, we'd find something good about each part—I began to see the wonder of my entire body. We also worked on self-esteem. It was an amazing change in my thinking, and that's how I gradually learned to accept myself as a whole.

I went into therapy because I wanted to know I was okay. I was so tired of hating myself and feeling like a second-class citizen. It was a time in my life when I took risks, and everything changed. Since then, I have continued to evolve. Al-

PROFILE

though I initially went into therapy to get help after the breakup of a relationship, it turned into a process of recovery and self-acceptance. The man I broke up with may have been the catalyst, and in a way I owe him a lot, but even more than that, I owe *me* a lot.

These days, I date up a storm. I've been in a number of relationships, but I haven't found anyone I want to spend the rest of my life with. When I was younger, I dated men who were attracted to *me* but not to big women; that was too hard for me to deal with. Now I only date men who like big women. And when I don't date, it's by choice; I've gone for several years without being in a relationship and felt fine about it. But there are times I feel the angst I think most women feel if they're almost 40 and single. Do I want to get married? That's a hard question to answer. Part of me—the part that wants the white dress and the happily-ever-after fairy tale—says yes. But the part of me that's strong and independent and doesn't want to answer to anybody says no. I'm often at odds with myself over this issue.

In terms of my health, I have no health problems of any sort. I get a physical every year to make sure I'm okay, and fortunately, I have a doctor who's not at all fat-phobic. He's been my G.P. since I was 18, and he never actively encourages me to lose weight—ever. He believes there's nothing medically wrong with me, and if my weight is discussed at all, it's because *I* bring it up. My only wish is that I could find a female ob-gyn who's fat-friendly. I haven't found one yet, but I keep looking.

I have a very active life. I go to a pool where, every Sunday, they have swimming for large-size women; I'm also trying to do more swimming during the week. Even though I don't like formal exercise, I'm on the go all the time. Besides my regular job, I have a small business on the side where I organize dances

PROFILE

for large-size people and their admirers. I have an active group of friends, and we're definitely out living life: we go to the movies, we travel on weekends . . . I'm not home a lot!

I believe that this country is slowly trying to accept fat people, but it's not there yet. Until recently, I was an active member of NAAFA [the National Association to Advance Fat Acceptance], and I would say that during the six years I was a member, I did see an improvement in the country's perceptions, but it's going to be a very long time before we're accepted by the majority of Americans. We still live in a very fat-phobic, "lookist" society. I also think much of the unwillingness to accept us has to do with economics; many groups simply don't want us to lose weight. Think about it: Therapists would make less money, the weight-loss industry would make less money . . . Dieting is a multi-billion-dollar industry. If there were fat acceptance in our society, some people would just lose too much of their income.

In the meantime, fat people get discriminated against every day of their lives. I've walked down the street and heard people tell me that I don't deserve to walk down the street because I'm fat and ugly. I've faced job discrimination, and I've been humiliated by potential employers. But you can't let it get you down. What works for me is to stare my oppressor in the face and speak up. For example, when I'm in the grocery store and I see someone looking to see what's in my cart, I make an effort to make eye contact with that person and look in their cart. If I'm in a restaurant and notice people staring at me or my fat friends, I stare back and sometimes I even say out loud, "Do you see them staring at us?"

Sitting back quietly is not acceptable to me. I used to avoid fighting back; I would just cower and let myself be a victim. I won't do that anymore. I believe most people who are prejudiced against fat people are ignorant and don't realize that their

PROFILE

taunts and anger hurt us. If we don't speak up and say, "It's not okay for you to do this," it will continue to happen. That's why I speak up every time.

What if you're still having trouble accepting yourself as you are? I urge you to go to that place that's buried deep inside of you and find that one little thing about your body that you like. Start telling yourself that you love that one little part. Maybe from there, you'll find another little part to love, and then another little part. Also, get angry! Stand up and say, "I'm not going to take this bad treatment anymore!" You have a right to be in this world. Take up your space!

CHAPTER EIGHT

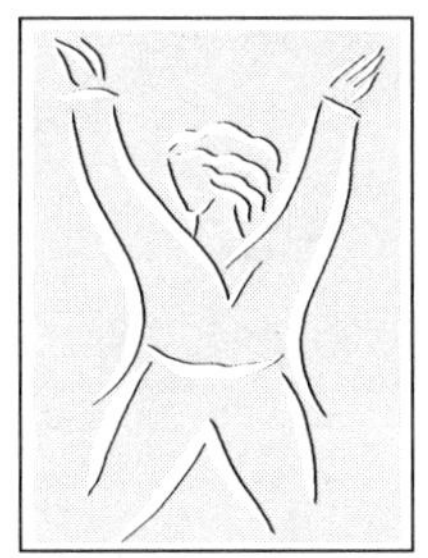

THE BIG PICTURE PLAN *for* HEALTH:

Smoking Cessation

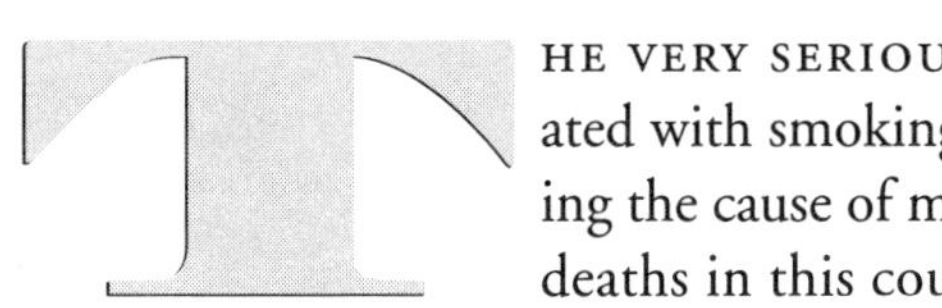

THE VERY SERIOUS HEALTH RISKS associated with smoking—beginning with its being the cause of more than 20 percent of all deaths in this country—have been known for several decades. While about half of all adults who have smoked have since quit, there are still too many smokers out there: 46 million, give or take a million. If you're among them, are you happy about it? Most of you aren't: 7 out of every 10 smokers in the U.S. today want to quit. Chances are, whatever pleasure you may derive from lighting up that cigarette, there's a part of you that probably feels more than a little concerned about it, knowing the damage it's doing to your health.

Once upon a time, we Americans tended to die from things like war and tuberculosis—events or plagues we had little or no personal control over. Sadly, these days more and more of us are dying—at least in part—from things we do to *ourselves.* In 1995, Dr. C. Everett Koop, former Surgeon General, told a group of health professionals in New York that the three top causes of death are 1) tobacco use; 2) harmful diet and activity patterns; and 3) excessive alcohol consumption. And if these unhealthy lifestyle habits don't sicken or kill you, they will, at the very least, make you poorer: preventable illness makes up 75 percent of our nation's financial medical burden.

Smoking As a Diet Aid?

If you're like many of America's 46 million smokers, you may well have picked up your first cigarette as a teenager (the time of life when virtually all smokers start) and used it as a food substitute, in the hopes of keeping your weight down. Think you came up with that idea yourself? Guess again. For nearly 75 years, cigarette companies have carefully *planned* to have you think that way.

You're probably too young to remember this, but back in the mid-1920s the advertising agency for Lucky Strike cigarettes came up with a brilliant scheme designed to lure female smokers—by making them think cigarettes were a fabulous diet aid. As the story goes, one day a Lucky Strike ad-agency honcho happened to see an overweight woman on the street—eating. Moments later, he spotted another woman who was slim, attractive—and smoking a cigarette. There and then, a marketing campaign was born.

It wasn't long before flappers were being seduced by ads for Lucky Strike depicting slender women and the slogan "Reach for a Lucky instead of a sweet." Did it work? You bet. By 1930, Luckys had gone from the third-bestselling brand in the country to number one. But if you think that since then we've all wised up enough to not fall for such ploys, think again. That marketing tactic has continued to be successful for such current-day brands as Virginia Slims and other slender cigarettes that subtly (or not so subtly) suggest slender bodies.

If you're reading this book, you may have learned the hard way that smoking is no guarantee that you won't overeat, nor is it a reliable "cure" for overweight. Even if smoking *does* keep your weight somewhat more manageable than it might be if you didn't smoke, that particular form of weight control comes at a very high price, as we'll explain later.

We know we don't need to lecture you about why you should quit smoking. You've read all the same health statistics we have. We take it for granted that you know smoking cigarettes causes a large number of major diseases. And you've surely noticed how more and more states have joined forces to sue cigarette manufacturers for the medical bills, paid for in part with state money, that are the result of smoking-related disease. But just in case you still doubt the wisdom of quitting smoking for the sake of your health—which is presumably why you're reading this book—we'd like to present you with a few eye-opening facts and figures:

- According to the Centers for Disease Control and Prevention (CDCP), tobacco use is the single most important preventable cause of death in the U.S., accounting for about one of every five deaths, or about 430,000 deaths annually.
- Cigarette smoking is a major causative risk factor for diseases of the heart and blood vessels; chronic bronchitis and emphysema; cancers of the lung, larynx, throat, mouth, esophagus, pancreas, and bladder; and diseases and negative health conditions such as respiratory infections, stomach ulcers, and others.
- Cigarette smoking is responsible for an estimated 21 percent of all coronary heart disease deaths (that number goes up to 40 percent in people under 65), 30 percent of all cancer deaths, and 87 percent of all lung cancer deaths in the U.S.
- The risk of dying from lung cancer is 22 times higher for men and 12 times higher for women who smoke compared with those who have never smoked.
- "Passive" smoking or "secondhand" smoke can cause lung cancer and other diseases in otherwise healthy adult nonsmokers and severe respiratory problems in children.
- Cigarette smoking during pregnancy is a risk factor for low birth weight, prematurity, miscarriage, sudden infant death syn-

drome (SIDS), and other health problems for mother and child. (Remarkably, despite all the health warnings, 25 percent of women still smoke throughout their pregnancy.)

• Cigarette smoking compounds the health risks of people whose work exposes them to hazardous chemical substances.

• Cigarette smoking makes you cough, as well as smell and taste like a dirty ashtray.

Need we go on?

Okay, now for the hard part. It's one thing to be alarmed about what cigarette smoking will do to your health; we know it's quite another to *do* something about it. We've been reading and hearing so much lately about the careful regulation of nicotine content by cigarette manufacturers, done deliberately in order to increase the likelihood of keeping their customers hooked. Manufacturers have known for years that most smokers don't smoke for the taste but because they are chemically addicted to nicotine. If you've ever tried to quit smoking in the past (and what smoker hasn't?), you always knew it was tough; now you have a lot more insight into the reasons *why* it's so tough. According to Elbert Glover, Ph.D., director of the Tobacco Research Center, smoking is more addictive today than ever—the average smoker smokes between 25 and 27 cigarettes per day.

So we won't kid you—if you're serious about giving up smoking for good, you have a difficult road ahead of you, although, interestingly enough, *not* as tough as the road to successful, long-term weight loss. Yes, you can do it! Indeed, the CDCP notes that cigarette smoking has declined dramatically since 1964, when the first Surgeon General's report on smoking appeared. In 1965, a whopping 42 percent of adults smoked; by 1992, that number had shrunk to 27 percent. And those who quit did themselves, and their health, a world of good: between 1965 and 1987 alone, 750,000 deaths were avoided or postponed, with approximately 20 years added to each quitter's life expectancy. Today, nearly half of all living adults who ever smoked have successfully stopped—and you can join their free-breathing ranks!

The question is, How *do* you quit for good?

Sending Your Cigarettes Up in Smoke

If you've ever tried to quit before, you may have had a host of reasons why you think you failed:

- "Oh, I wasn't really into it."
- "There were too many things going on in my life, and quitting smoking wasn't something I could focus on."
- "I was having all those financial problems. I *needed* to smoke to deal with the stress."
- "I like how calm smoking makes me feel."
- "My smoking-cessation program was going great, but then my son had that terrible accident, and I just started smoking again."
- "What can I say? I'm hooked on nicotine!"

And the list goes on and on.

Whatever your reasons for not succeeding before—and no matter how many times you quit and then resumed smoking—the good news is that **you can still quit permanently**. If you're reading this book, you're probably highly motivated to improve your health. That's great, because mobilizing your motivation is one of the three keys to your cigarette-kicking success. The other two are *commitment* and *planning*.

You've got to *want* to quit this time to the point where you're willing to make the commitment to this all-important health goal and, even more important, to yourself. Furthermore, you've got to have a *plan*—one that not only encompasses the step-by-steps for quitting, but also helps you handle stressful situations and negative moods as they arise without using cigarettes. You're *not* going to do that anymore.

You're going to have a concrete plan that will help see you through the ups and downs—because you and your health are worth it. While some people *do* manage to kick smoking by quitting cold turkey, planning a course of action that you'll be following over a period of weeks—as well as putting in place healthy alternatives when you feel you "must" have a cigarette—is a more effective strategy for the vast majority of smokers. We're going to show you how to create such a plan for yourself.

Quitting for Good: The How-Tos

We suggest that, before you proceed, you go back to Chapter Four, which discusses the six stages of change in any lifestyle behavior. Reviewing the points in that chapter will help you determine whether you are indeed at the right stage of your life to quit smoking permanently (and, if not, when in the future you might be better equipped, mentally and physically, to take on this project).

The smoking-cessation tips you see here come from those who know, experts at the National Cancer Institute:

Preparing Yourself for Quitting

• Decide positively that you want to quit. Try to avoid negative thoughts about how difficult it might be.

• List all the reasons you want to quit. Every night before going to bed, say one of those reasons to yourself 10 times.

• Think about the other strong personal reasons there are for quitting, in addition to benefiting your health and satisfying your obligations to friends and family. For example, think of all the money you spend on cigarettes, all the time you waste taking cigarette breaks, rushing out to buy a pack, hunting for a light, trying to get rid of the yellow stains on your teeth and fingers, alleviating the staleness of your breath, regretting the loss of taste for healthy food, and so on.

• Begin to condition yourself physically: start a modest exercise program, drink more fluids, get plenty of rest, and avoid fatigue.

• Set a target date for quitting—perhaps a special day such as your birthday, your wedding anniversary, or the Great American Smokeout day (the third Thursday in November). If you smoke heavily at work, start your quitting program during your vacation so that you're already committed to quitting when you return. Make the date sacred; don't let anything change it. This will make it easier for you to keep track of the day you became a nonsmoker, and it will give you one more special occasion to celebrate every year!

Knowing What to Expect

• Have realistic expectations. Quitting isn't easy, but it's not impossible either. More than 3 million Americans (about 8,000 per day) quit smoking every year.

• Understand that withdrawal symptoms are temporary. They usually last only one to two weeks.

• Know that most relapses occur in the first week after quitting, when withdrawal symptoms are strongest and your body is still dependent on nicotine. Be aware that this will be your hardest time. Use all your personal resources—willpower, family, friends, the information here—to get you through this critical period.

Involving Others

• Ask a friend or spouse to quit with you.

• Tell your family and friends that you're quitting, and when. They can be an important source of support both before and after you quit.

• Bet a friend that you can quit on your target date. Put your cigarette money aside for every day you don't smoke, and forfeit it to the friend if you do smoke. (But if you do go back to smoking, *don't give up*. Simply strengthen your resolve and try again.)

Ways of Quitting

Switch Brands

• Switch to a brand you don't like.

• Change to a brand that's low in tar and nicotine a couple of weeks before your target date. However, *do not* smoke more cigarettes, inhale them more often or more deeply, or place your fingertips over the holes in the filters (which increases the total amount of nicotine you take in). Your goal is to cut down gradually on your daily nicotine dose. That's the reason for switching brands in the first place.

Gradually Reduce the Number of Cigarettes You Smoke Each Day

• At the beginning, smoke the same number of cigarettes as before but only *half* of each one (or even half of every other one).

• Each day, postpone the lighting of your first cigarette by one hour (or a half-hour).

• Decide you'll smoke only during odd or even hours of the day or only before or after certain hours.

• Decide beforehand how many cigarettes you'll smoke each day. For each additional cigarette you smoke, give a dollar to your favorite charity. (Some people give their cigarette money to an organization or individual they *don't* like or respect, to help get them back on track that much sooner.)

• Change your smoking and eating habits. For example, drink milk when you smoke, which many people consider incompatible with smoking. Eat foods at the end of your meals that won't automatically lead you to a cigarette.

• Remember: Cutting down can help you quit but it's not a substitute for quitting. Once you're down to about seven cigarettes a day, it's time to set your target date to quit and get ready to stick to it.

Don't Smoke Automatically

• Take note of the mental and physical associations you have with each cigarette you smoke. Smoke only those cigarettes you *really* want or need. Catch yourself before you light up a cigarette out of pure habit.

• If you find associations with certain behaviors, try deliberately to break one or more. For example, tell yourself, "I'm going to stop smoking cigarettes when I'm drinking coffee" or "when talking on the phone," etc.

• Don't empty your ashtrays. This will remind you of how many cigarettes you've smoked each day, and the sight and smell of the stale cigarette butts may well turn you off.

• Make yourself aware of each cigarette: use the opposite hand for holding it, or put your cigarette pack into a different pocket or an unfamiliar location to break the automatic reach.

Make Smoking Inconvenient

• Stop buying cigarettes by the carton. Wait until one pack is empty before you buy another.

• Stop carrying cigarettes with you. Make them difficult to get.

Make Smoking Unpleasant

• If you like to smoke with others, smoke alone. Turn your chair toward an empty corner, focusing only on the cigarette (and how unhealthy it is).

• Collect all your cigarette butts in one large glass container as a visual reminder of the filth created by smoking.

Just Before Quitting

• Practice going without cigarettes for increasingly longer stretches of time.

• Don't think of *never* smoking again. Think of quitting in terms of one day at a time.

• When you wake up in the morning, tell yourself that you won't smoke today—then don't.

• Wash or dry-clean your clothes to rid them of the cigarette smell.

On the Day You Quit

• Throw away all your cigarettes and matches. Hide your lighters and ashtrays.

• Keep very busy. Go to the movies (consider a double feature), take a long walk, go bike riding, go to the beach.

• Remind your family and friends that this is your quit date, and ask them to be prepared to help you over the rough spots of the first few days and weeks.

• Buy yourself a treat or do something special to celebrate.

• Go to the dentist to have your teeth cleaned, to get rid of the tobacco stains. Notice how nice your teeth look and resolve to keep them that way.

• Make a list of things you'd like to buy for yourself or someone else. Estimate the cost in terms of packs of cigarettes, and put the money aside to buy those presents.

Immediately After Quitting

• Create a clean, fresh, nonsmoking environment around yourself at work and at home. Buy yourself flowers. (You may be surprised how much you can enjoy their scent now.)

• The first few days after you quit, spend as much time as possible in places where smoking isn't allowed—libraries, museums, department stores, theaters, public conveyances, houses of worship.

• Drink large quantities of water and fruit juice. Avoid alcohol and caffeinated beverages, such as coffee, which you might associate with smoking.

• If you miss the sensation of having something in your hand, hold a pencil or a paper clip.

• If you miss having something in your mouth, try sugarless gum, toothpicks, or a fake cigarette.

Avoid Temptation

• Instead of reaching for a cigarette after a meal, get up from the table and brush your teeth or go for a walk.

• If you always smoke while driving, listen to a particularly interesting radio program or your favorite music, or take public transportation for a while, if you can.

• For the first few weeks, avoid situations you strongly associate with the pleasurable aspects of smoking, such as watching your favorite television show, sitting in your favorite chair, or having a cocktail before dinner.

• Until you are confident of your ability to stay off cigarettes, limit your socializing to healthful and/or outdoor activities or situations where smoking isn't permitted.

Find New Habits

• Change your habits to make smoking difficult, unpleasant, or unnecessary. For example, it's hard to smoke when you're running, playing handball, or lifting weights. Do things that require the use of your hands—gardening, needlework, letter writing, crossword puzzles. Take the dog for a walk. Give yourself a manicure.

• Stretch a lot. Move your body more often.

• Get plenty of rest.

• Pay attention to your appearance. Put some of that money you've saved by not buying cigarettes toward a new haircut or outfit.

When You Get the Crazies

• Keep (healthy) oral substitutes handy—carrots, sunflower seeds, apples, celery, raisins, sugarless gum.

• Rinse your mouth with mouthwash. Brush your teeth. Remind yourself how nice your mouth feels this way.

• Take 10 deep breaths and hold the last one while lighting a match. Exhale slowly and blow out the match. Pretend it's a cigarette and crush it out in an ashtray.

• If possible, take a shower or bath.

• Relax. (See Chapter Seven on deep breathing and other stress-reduction techniques.)

• Never allow yourself to think, "Just one cigarette won't hurt." It will.

What You Can Look Forward To

YES, YOU CAN FOCUS on how much you'll really miss that morning cigarette with your coffee or that afternoon smoke break you always took at work. It will be tough at first. But very soon after you quit, a lot of wonderful things will happen to you:

• Within 12 hours after having your last cigarette, your body will begin to heal itself. Levels of carbon monoxide and nicotine in your system will decline rapidly. Your heart and lungs will begin to repair the damage caused by cigarette smoke.

• Within days, your senses of smell and taste will most likely improve.

• You'll breathe more easily.

• You may continue to cough for a while, but that unpleasant cougher's hack that used to annoy all those movie patrons and co-workers will start to disappear.

• You will no longer have to worry about setting your house on fire by smoking in bed.

• You can now answer personal ads that say, "Nonsmokers only need apply."

• You will be free of the mess, the smell, the inconvenience, the expense, and the physical and psychological dependence on smoking. Perhaps best of all, your health-risk level will soon begin returning to normal.

True, you may have to go through an unpleasant phase before some of the benefits kick in. For example, some people may experience one or more of the following once they stop smoking: dry mouth, increased hunger, irritability, sleep problems, headaches, and, yes, cigarette cravings, which can be quite strong. Hang in there. Deal with these situations appropriately as they arise (if you feel tired, take a nap; if you feel hungry, have a sensible snack) without automatically reaching for a cigarette. Remember, these symptoms are the results of your body clearing out the nicotine, *a powerful addictive chemical.* But the good news is that most of the nicotine should be out of your system within two or three days.

Congratulations (But Keep Your Guard Up)

WHETHER IT'S BEEN TWO WEEKS or two months since your last smoke, the point is, you've made it through. But your work isn't done yet. You know as well as we do that temptations lurk around every corner, whether it's in the form of a bar in full Happy Hour swing, a buddy who smokes and urges you to join him "just this once," or that post-dinner cup of coffee *begging* for a cigarette to accompany it. Instead of giving in to the next urge to smoke that comes your way, you must instantly remind yourself that you are now in a new category: *nonsmoker.* That is a status of which you can be very proud. You do not smoke anymore.

As you resist each urge, use your success as a learning experience. Ask yourself:

- Where was I when I got the urge?
- What was I doing at the time?
- Who was with me?
- What was I thinking/feeling?
- What did I do to get through it—what was the secret of my success in controlling the urge?

Stay on guard for vulnerable moments and situations that would normally lead you to reach for a cigarette. Sometimes you *will* be in one of those situations. (You can't be out playing handball all the time.) It's a good idea to make a list of your typical smoking triggers, so you can anticipate them and be prepared with an alternate activity. Your smoking triggers may include:

- feeling under pressure at work
- feeling blue
- having an alcoholic drink or a cup of coffee
- driving
- watching television
- watching someone else smoke

Have your list of alternative activities at the ready so that when temptation strikes, you'll be prepared. Whether your favorite fall-back activity is exercising, calling a good friend, 5 or 10 minutes of meditation or progressive muscle relaxation (see Chapter Seven on stress management), buying yourself a small gift for your accomplishment to date, or simply basking in the glory of being an ex-smoker, do it! The more you use your coping skills, the stronger you get and the more easily you'll be able to resist temptation the next time around.

If You're Still Afraid You'll Put On Weight If You Quit Smoking

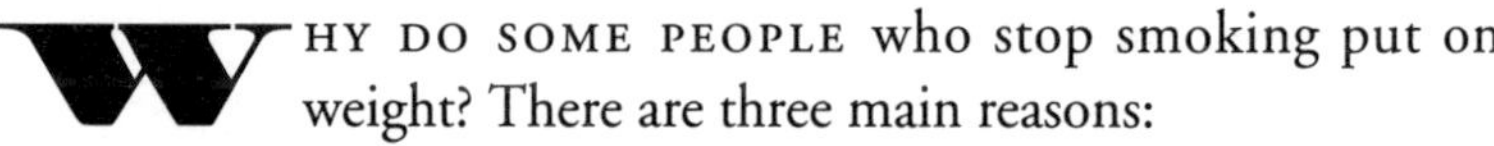

WHY DO SOME PEOPLE who stop smoking put on weight? There are three main reasons:

1. You need/want something to do with your mouth and fingers, and you may eat more than before.

2. The nicotine in cigarettes suppresses the body's insulin levels. Insulin is the hormone that helps your body use sugar and keeps your sweet tooth at bay. When smokers quit, they often find that they now crave cookies and cake—not to mention more food in general, which suddenly tastes much better than it used to because, without tobacco, their taste buds have sprung to life.

3. Nicotine speeds up your metabolism, so when it's no longer present in your system, the calories you normally consume may not be burned as efficiently.

However, the smoking/weight relationship is not nearly as bad as people imagine. A study published in the November 2, 1995, issue of *The New England Journal of Medicine* examined the influence of smoking cessation on weight gain. Between 1978 and 1990, the percentage of Americans who gained weight increased markedly while the percentage of smokers dropped markedly, initially leading the researchers to consider the possibility that there was some connection between the two—namely, that quitting smoking automatically led to weight gain. And indeed, for many of those studied, there *was* a weight gain over the length of the 10-year study—*but of only about 10 pounds per person.* Not much of a gain. Also, as the study was quick to add, "The health benefits of smoking cessation far exceed the risks associated with weight gain." In fact, according to some estimates, you'd have to gain *100 to 150 pounds* after you quit smoking for your weight-related health risks to equal your smoking-related health risks. Furthermore, as the study went on to say, "The health benefits of smoking cessation are undeniable," while, as we've noted a number of times in this book, though there are a number of benefits associated with weight loss, unless you are significantly overweight, improvement of your health status is not one of them.

Sure, you don't want to worry about weight gain after you've accomplished the very impressive task of quitting smoking. That is why the researchers urge anyone who quits smoking and *does* happen to put on those 10-odd pounds to "attempt to limit further weight gain." That's something you can do by being especially careful of the snacks you eat (as we've said, you're likely to want to nibble more, particularly in the early stages of your smoking-cessation program) and/or increasing your exercise. Keep your weight steady, keep those cigarettes out of sight, and you'll be amazed at how good you feel.

More Tips to Help You Quit

• Don't get discouraged if you don't succeed right away. Relapse is considered a normal part of the smoking-cessation process and only brings you closer to quitting permanently. The average cigarette quitter relapses three or four times before quitting for good. View any relapse you might have as a learning experience, and try again. Remember, about half of all adults who ever smoked are now ex-smokers, even if it took many of them several tries to get there.

• Keep in mind that a method that works for your spouse or your co-worker may not work for you. Try different smoking-cessation techniques until you find one you're comfortable with.

• Nicotine replacement therapy (NRT), including patches and gum (now available without prescription), has proven very effective, although this method can be costly. According to the "Smoking Cessation Clinical Practice Guideline Consensus Statement," published in the April 24, 1996, issue of the *Journal of the American Medical Association*, "[Our] panel identified nicotine replacement therapy (nicotine patches and nicotine gum) as the only pharmacotherapy currently shown to be effective as an aid to smoking cessation. The panel recommends that, unless there is a clear medical contraindication, all patients planning a quit attempt should be offered nicotine replacement therapy." You may want to discuss with your health-care provider whether such a course of treatment is a good idea for you.

• If you're having a hard time trying to quit on your own, you may want to get support from a local smoking-cessation workshop or program. You may find the name of one through your health plan or local hospital or from your health-care provider. Or call 1-800-LUNG-USA, the American Lung Association's number, or 1-800-4-CANCER, the National Cancer Institute's Cancer Information Service. Those programs that tend to be most helpful address a variety of smoking-related issues, including physical and psychological addiction, weight control, overall health, and stress management.

• Constantly remind yourself how important this goal is for you *and* for your family. Not only do you want to protect the ones you love from the ill effects of your secondhand smoke, but you want to be around them—and in good health—for as long as you possibly can.

PROFILE

Dee Links

Columbus, Ohio
Age: 39
Height: 5'2"
Weight: 299 pounds
Occupation: Manager of the CompuServe "Ample Living" On-Line Forum

EXCEPT FOR MY BROTHER, everyone on both sides of my family is large, especially the women. We're all around 5' tall and over 300 pounds. I was put on my first diet at age 5. By the time I was 10, I was addicted to amphetamines. Until my early 20s, my weight went up and down. I did every diet known to mankind: the Atkins diet, the grapefruit diet, everything. It was always the same: As soon as I'd go off the diet, I would gain the weight back and then some—immediately. The very last diet I went on was Optifast. Right after I came off it, I developed gallstones and had to have surgery. (I found out later that gallstones could be a side effect of that diet.) Back then, they didn't have the laparoscopic procedure they have now, so I have a big scar from the midpoint of my stomach all the way to my right hip.

I decided then and there that, since I wasn't getting permanent results, it was ridiculous to continually do these things to my body. So at age 23, weighing 290 pounds, I decided I'd had enough. No more dieting. I didn't know what would happen to my weight; I only knew that dieting had made me fatter. To my surprise, my weight pretty much stabilized after that. Now I fluctuate only about 5 to 10 pounds, depending on the time of year and how active I am. In the summer, for ex-

Profile

ample, I garden a lot and I'm generally more active, so I usually weigh a little less.

From my teens on, I've always been an emotional eater—I would eat whenever I was feeling stressed or depressed. But now I eat in a healthier way; my emotional eating is under control. I keep my fat intake to 30 grams a day or less—I read nutrition labels big time! I also try to eat a high-fiber diet—I have chronic colitis, and the fiber helps control it. Otherwise, I have no health problems. My family has a history of high blood pressure, diabetes, and heart disease, but not me, even though I'm overweight. I guess it's because I eat a healthy diet and exercise regularly. I *had* been on medication for blood pressure, but when I quit smoking five months ago, my blood pressure dropped. Now I'm off the medication. My whole family used to smoke, but they quit after my mother died of a heart attack six years ago. What helped me give up cigarettes was realizing that I didn't have to go down the same path my mother did—I could quit now! The same thing with exercise. She never exercised, but I do.

Since I quit smoking, I've actually *lost* weight! I was 308 pounds when I quit, and when I weighed myself three weeks ago, I was 299. Every time I got the urge for a cigarette, I would get on my treadmill or go out for a walk instead. I exercise daily—20 minutes on a treadmill. That's my thing; I've been doing it for two years. I do it because I care about being fit and mobile, *not* because I care about being thin.

I've been married for five years. My husband, Alan, is tall and slender—we're like Mutt and Jeff! When Alan asked me out, it was love at first sight for both of us. I weighed between 290 and 300 pounds when we were dating, but my weight was not a problem. In fact, I've never had problems with men regarding my weight. I've had an active social life since I was 18 or 19. I know that goes against society's idea that a woman

PROFILE

needs to be thin to get a man. My own mother said I'd never get married because no man would want a fat girl. I proved her wrong! Alan and I are very happily married. He finds me very attractive and sexy—he frequently brings me home sexy teddies and lacy bras. Ladies, you can get *your* man to do the same thing. Just point him in the direction of the right stores!

I started the "Ample Living" Forum on CompuServe. A lot of the reason was to try to give back to other people some of what I've learned, namely, that the window dressing doesn't matter. It's what's inside that counts, whether you weigh 100 pounds or 900 pounds.

When you're comfortable with yourself, then the looks and stares of other people will no longer bother you; you will no longer use them to form your opinion of yourself or your self-worth. The blatant comments are much harder to avoid, of course, but this is what I do when I hear one: I go right up to the person's face, look him in the eye, and tell him I'm suffering from a horrible cancer that's killing me, that I'm on a steroid that makes me fat, and that I'll be dead in three months anyway, so he won't have to worry about me anymore! Yes, I have chutzpah! I do this on purpose because I want these people to think twice before they talk that way to the next fat person.

If you choose to do something about your weight, do it as a lifestyle change, not as a short-term diet. Diets don't work—that's been proven over and over. If you do try to lose weight, do it for the purpose of improving your health, not to fit into society better. Love yourself—really, it's the only way to live.

PROFILE

Pat Carroll

Cape Cod, Massachusetts
Age: 68
Height: 5'3"
Weight: "Just under 200 pounds"
Occupation: Actress and singer

MY WEIGHT HAS GONE UP AND DOWN over the years, ever since I was 8 years old. It's a familial problem—my mother and grandmother both had weight problems all their lives. My experiences with weight seem to prove that it's not always a matter of food; if you have family that runs toward fat, you probably will too. I was always active as a kid—I was an almost-daily tennis player and swimmer—so my weight was solid; I was a muscular person because I was always using my muscles. I haven't been very athletic recently, so I *feel* my weight more—I actually feel the flesh on my body because I'm not using it the way I used to. But I still try to swim as much as I can.

In the past two years, I've also been concentrating on a low-fat food program, mostly to lower my cholesterol. I'm doing it for another reason: I have to have knee-replacement surgery, and my doctor suggested it would be better both before and after the surgery if I had about 50 pounds off me. I started my food program weighing 220 pounds. I haven't weighed myself in about a year, but I've gone down two sizes. I haven't set a date for surgery yet, but sometime during the next year, I'll step on a scale, and if I see I've lost 50 pounds, I'll book the surgery. Then again, maybe I won't, not if I feel wonderful!

I don't wear a halo about following my food program. I

PROFILE

will occasionally have a happy fling, and when I do, I don't feel guilty about it. I feel satisfied with my food plan. My diet includes many of the foods I *like* to eat—when I changed my way of eating, I decided I wasn't going to let myself feel deprived.

I also stopped smoking in the last two months, which, fortunately, hasn't made me go too crazy with food. Quitting smoking has not only improved my health, but now I'm also able to sustain notes longer when I sing, and my speaking voice is not so saloonish. That, in my profession, is a lovely plus.

In my mind and my body, I know what I need to keep me going. On this low-fat diet, I find I have loads of energy, which I need at my age because I'm still working johnny-be-deviled. When you're younger, you usually have a surplus of energy, and it's okay if you sometimes overextend yourself, but I can't do that now; I must be very careful. For example, if one week I have daily rehearsals for a show, I must really look at my entire week and say, When will I rest? Rest is very important for me—if I get enough sleep, I can face anything. And I must also ask myself, When will I fit in a bit of exercise, even if it's just a walk around the block, without dipping into my energy savings account? That's the best thing that has happened to my thinking lately: realizing the importance of maintaining a balance in my life, so I don't have to knock my brains out to keep functioning at a good level.

I think older people today have the attitude, "I don't care what I look like as long as I feel good, I'm living life to the fullest, and I'm staying in balance." I must admit it still shocks me that I have white hair! But that doesn't make a difference as long as I feel good. The real questions are: Are you comfortable? Do you feel good in your clothes? Do you look in the mirror and like the person you see there? Is that a person you'd like to talk to? It's not enough to just look in the mir-

PROFILE

ror; what's important is how you feel about the image reflected back to you.

I can't change the perception society has of me, but I *can* change my perception of myself, and the way I do that best is through my work. I'm doing more things I've never done before, and I'm taking more risks. I'm going to do a Ben Jonson play for the first time, and I'm playing Volpone—a man. I've played men before—I was Falstaff in a production of *The Merry Wives of Windsor*—and to me, it's very exciting that, at my age, I've been able to work in classical theater and achieve a modicum of success doing it. You can find great joy in the discovery of new things, and it's wonderful when your work does that for you.

I don't care what age you are or what reason you have to do it, but if we're all being told to get on the wonderful bandwagon of health, then we should. We know cigarette smoking isn't good for our health, so, okay, cut it out. We know we need some fat in our diet, so you don't cut it out totally—you keep some. The Greeks said, "Moderation in all things," and if you use that as your guide, you can't fall far from any mark you set for yourself.

Chapter Nine

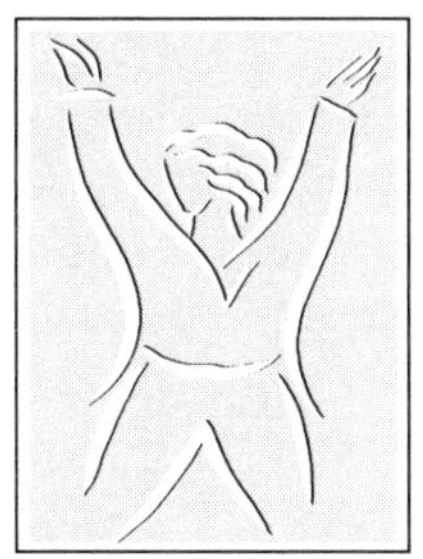

The Big Picture Plan *for* Health:

Personal Safety

Do you think that being a healthy person only means eating right, exercising regularly, and tossing that pack of cigarettes into the trash? Think again. Living a long, rewarding life *also* means consciously protecting yourself from physical harm, keeping an eye out for your personal safety as much as you would that of a small child or an ill person in your care. In a way, it seems like obvious advice. Yet we all know someone who never buckles her seat belt (although she might be able to tell you the precise number of fat grams on her plate at any given moment) or that George Hamilton wannabe who, despite all the skin-cancer warnings, continues to worship the sun (after slathering on only baby oil).

As we mentioned earlier, with the eradication in the last century of many of the worst diseases known to mankind, we should, as a nation, be enjoying greater health and longevity than ever before. And, to an extent, we are. But as with the health problems we bring upon ourselves through poor eating habits, physical inactivity, and unmanaged stress, we've cooked up still *other* ways to harm the health and shorten the lives of ourselves and our loved ones—by being careless about our safety in and out of the home. Who among us, while watching the horrifying sight on the evening news of a house going up in flames or a car driver dead following a head-on collision, believes it can ever happen to us? And yet we know all too well that it can. Indeed, up to 1 in 20 deaths in our country is the result of personal injury, whether at home, outdoors, or on the job.

However, you should know that a very large percentage of these deaths could have been prevented. There is much you can do to lower your risk of such calamities. Further, for the overweight person intent upon improving her overall health, taking steps toward personal safety, such as those outlined below, may be among the easiest first steps to take.

Think about it. Once you get into the habit of buckling your seat belt every time you get in the car, or taking the time to install fire extinguishers in the proper locations around your house, isn't it possible that you may slowly develop the discipline to start working on making those tougher lifestyle changes, such as exercising regularly and quitting smoking? We're secretly hoping that by following the personal-safety suggestions in this chapter, you will wind up getting a *double* benefit—both the personal-safety behavior change itself *and* the other positive changes it might lead you to later on.

On the following pages are some simple ways to stay safe and sound—in your home, in your car, and in the sun.

At-Home Safety Checklist

As the National Safety Council points out, the right answers to these questions that they have developed can keep you and your family safe from harm at home.

In the Kitchen . . .

Do you have a special rack or compartment for storing sharp knives, rather than just keeping them in a drawer?

Yes_____ No_____

Do you store kitchen matches in a tightly closed metal container?

Yes_____ No_____

Do you wipe or pick up spilled water, grease, or food peelings immediately so you won't slip and fall?

Yes_____ No_____

Do you dry your hands before using an electrical appliance, to significantly lower your risk of getting a shock?

Yes_____ No_____

Do you wear short sleeves while cooking? (Long sleeves can catch fire or snag on the handles of cookware.)

Yes_____ No_____

Do you keep a close watch on food cooking on the stove?

Yes_____ No_____

Do you use pot holders or oven mitts?

Yes_____ No_____

Do you use microwave-safe containers for microwave cooking?

Yes_____ No_____

Do you shield yourself from scalding steam when you lift the lids from hot pans and microwave containers? (Lift the far side of the lid first.)

Yes_____ No_____

Do you turn pot handles away from the front of the stove and from other burners, to keep them from getting too hot to handle?

Yes_____ No_____

Do you keep oven and broiler pans free of grease?

Yes_____ No_____

Are you careful not to throw water on a grease fire, which will only spread the fire?

Yes_____ No_____

Do you keep a pot lid near the stove to smother flames from a grease fire? (*Immediately* turn off the burner too.)

Yes_____ No_____

Do you keep a fire extinguisher in your kitchen?

Yes_____ No_____

Is your kitchen wiring appropriate for the load drawn by your electrical appliances and oven?

Yes_____ No_____

In the Bathroom . . .

Does your tub or shower have a slip-resistant surface?

Yes_____ No_____

If you have grab bars, are they securely fastened?

Yes_____ No_____

Do bathroom mats have slip-resistant backing?

Yes_____ No_____

Are medicines clearly labeled?

Yes_____ No_____

Do you throw away any medications that are past their expiration date?

Yes_____ No_____

If there are young children at home, do you buy childproof medicine containers and keep them stored in locked cabinets where they can't be reached by youngsters?

Yes_____ No_____

Do you store breakable bottles and jars where they can't be shattered?

Yes_____ No_____

Are there night-lights in the bathroom for young children and elderly relatives?

Yes_____ No_____

Do you unplug electrical appliances when not in use to reduce the chance of shock?

Yes_____ No_____

In the Bedroom . . .

Do the smokers in the family avoid smoking in bed? (Smoking in bed is one of the most common causes of both fatal and nonfatal house fires.)

Yes_____ No_____

Is there a *working* smoke detector in every bedroom?

Yes_____ No_____

Are there night-lights in the bedroom for young children and elderly relatives? Are they at a safe distance from bedding, curtains, or other materials that could catch fire?

Yes_____ No_____

Do you avoid walking in your stocking feet on smooth floors? (Falls are one of the most common causes of injury and even death, especially for the elderly.)

Yes_____ No_____

In the Halls and on Stairways . . .

Are the stairs and hallways clearly lighted? Are there switches at the top and bottom of the stairways?

Yes_____ No_____

Do all steps and stairways have a sturdy handrail on both sides?

Yes_____ No_____

Do you keep stairways free of any objects and is stairway carpeting free of tears or protruding nails?

Yes_____ No_____

Are exits and passageways kept free of boxes, furniture, toys, and other obstructions?

Yes_____ No_____

Do small rugs have slip-resistant backing?

Yes_____ No_____

All Around the House . . .

Do you keep a list of emergency phone numbers (police, fire, doctor, poison-control center, local utilities) next to each phone?

Yes_____ No_____

Do you keep the instruction manuals for your appliances so you can check if something goes wrong?

Yes_____ No_____

Does everyone in the family know where the emergency shut-offs are located for electric, gas, and water service, and for the furnace?

Yes_____ No_____

Do you avoid overloading electrical outlets, another common cause of house fires?

Yes_____ No_____

Do you keep a working flashlight in a convenient location?

Yes_____ No_____

Do you check smoke-detector batteries every month and replace them every year?

Yes_____ No_____

Do you keep fire extinguishers inspected and recharged when necessary? Do family members know when and how to use them?

Yes_____ No_____

Do you avoid running electrical cords under carpeting or hanging them from nails?

Yes_____ No_____

Do you get help for heavy or difficult jobs to reduce your risk of injury and particularly back strain?

Yes_____ No_____

Does your family have a home escape plan in case of fire? Do you go through a practice drill every six months?

Yes_____ No_____

Sun Sense

WITH A SIGH, you've given in to the warnings. You've finally stopped lying on your roof or in your backyard, dripping with oil and gripping the sun reflector around your face so you can get "a little color." And, okay, so you still go to the beach occasionally when the temperature soars and the sun and surf beckon—but it's not the morning-till-night fry-fest it was in your youth.

It's a start.

The effects of the sun are powerful and potentially dangerous to our health, even when we take precautions. The American Cancer Society reports that skin cancer is currently the most common type of cancer—more than 800,000 of us get one of the three most common types each year. The good news is that, when caught early, skin cancer can usually be cured. The bad news is that we still have to be on guard much of the time.

Who is likely to get skin cancer?

If you fall into one of these categories, you're at greater-than-average risk for developing skin cancer:

- fair-skinned
- redheaded or blonde
- sunburn easily
- spend a lot of time in the sun

As you might imagine, those parts of your body that are normally uncovered are where some 90 percent of skin cancers will develop: the face, hands, forearms, and ears.

How do you prevent skin cancer?

The best answer is also the most obvious: Stay out of the sun. But if you *must* be outdoors for extended periods of time, at least take these precautions:

- Avoid the sun when the rays are strongest, from 10 A.M. until 3 P.M.
- Cover up. Wear wide-brimmed hats, long-sleeved shirts and pants. Keep your neck covered, too, with a collar or a loose-fitting scarf.

• Use sunscreen with an SPF (sun protection factor) of at least 15. Apply it at least 15 to 30 minutes before going into the sun, and reapply it after swimming or sweating. If you wear liquid foundation makeup, look for the type that has sunscreen in it.

• Beware of cloudy days and sunny winter days—you can still get burned at these times.

• The sun's rays can reach through three feet of water, so be careful even if you're in a pool or the ocean.

Another tip: Avoid sunlamps, tanning parlors, and tanning pills, all of which can be as harmful as the sun.

Also, routinely check your skin for anything out of the ordinary. Check moles, spots, and birthmarks every month for any changes.

How can you tell if you might have skin cancer?

• a mole changes size, shape, or color

• there is an unusual growth on your skin

• a sore won't heal

• you develop red, scaly patches on your skin (they can become cancerous)

If you see any of these conditions, visit your doctor as soon as possible.

Safe-Driving Basics

In 1995, there were 177 million of us licensed drivers on the road—enough to cause a lot of damage. Some 43,900 folks lost their lives in auto accidents that year, while more than two million suffered disabling injuries while in a moving vehicle. Since your health and longevity are of primary concern to you, you've got to be a smart driver (*and* passenger). Follow these rules of the road from the National Safety Council:

Wear your seat belt. And make sure those in your car do the same. Believe it or not, it's estimated that only 46 percent of drivers buckle up. According to the National Highway Traffic Safety Administration, when lap and shoulder safety belts are used, they reduce the risk of fatal injury to front-seat passengers by 45 percent and the risk of moderate to critical injury by 50 percent.

Don't drink and drive. If you plan to drink, be sure to designate a driver who won't. Alcohol is a factor in almost half of all fatal motor vehicle accidents.

Don't exceed the speed limit. Speeding is a factor in about one-third of all vehicle crash fatalities. (In a collision, the chance that you will be fatally injured doubles with each 10 miles of speed over 50 mph that the car is traveling.)

Don't let yourself get too tired while driving. If you're taking a long car trip, allow yourself enough time to take frequent breaks for a light snack or to stretch. The moment you find yourself driving while drowsy, STOP and get some rest before continuing.

Drive defensively. Be alert to drivers who are driving dangerously or erratically. Keep a good distance between you and the vehicle in front of you.

Don't let your car phone be the cause of an accident. The safest type of car phone is a cellular phone with a hands-free speakerphone option, with the microphone installed in the sun visor directly above the driver's line of vision. The handset should be easily accessible, allowing you to sit and drive normally while you talk on the phone. Avoid dialing while the car is in motion. Always keep both hands on the steering wheel and eyes on the road, using the speakerphone and leaving the handset in its cradle whenever the car is moving. Remember, your first consideration at all times while driving should be *driving*, not talking on the phone.

Always keep the following items in your car in case of a breakdown or other emergency:

- a jack
- a spare tire
- a ⅜"-to-1"-thick plywood board to support the jack
- a lug wrench
- screwdrivers (Phillips and flat head)
- a flashlight
- fuses
- a fire extinguisher
- flares and/or reflective triangles

- jumper cables
- engine fluids such as oil and coolant
- a first-aid kit

Making these personal-safety changes may all seem quite simple—even simplistic. But particularly if you've had trouble in the past launching or maintaining a positive lifestyle change, starting with something simple may be just the ticket. What better way to prove to yourself that you *can* take steps to improve your health than by making some of the small-yet-significant changes recommended here? After this, who knows how much you can accomplish?

PROFILE

Camryn Manheim

New York, New York
Age: 35
Height: 5'10"
Weight: 250 pounds
Occupation: Actor/playwright/teacher/ sign-language interpreter

I'VE ALWAYS HAD A PREDISPOSITION to being overweight—it's been a struggle for everyone in my immediate *and* my extended family. I was an active, fairly normal child from Peoria, Illinois. I started gaining weight for the first time at about age 10, when my family moved to southern California. The most surprising thing to me about California was that people shopped for their groceries in bikinis! The two most terrifying things you could do—shopping for food and being practically naked—they would do together! So, in an effort to not have to wear a bathing suit to school, I rebelled and got fat.

I had a compulsive-eating problem. I'd steal money from my mother's purse and buy outrageous amounts of candy. When I wasn't eating candy, I'd be thinking about candy and how to get the money to buy it. As I got older, I kept getting heavier. Then, when I was 23 and in graduate school, I was told I'd have to lose weight; otherwise I would be jeopardizing my standing in the school. I was studying drama, and the teachers felt that losing weight would be indicative of my commitment to myself as an artist and to my body as an instrument—you know how they're always telling actors that Your Body Is Your Instrument. Also, they felt that losing weight would help me psychologically and emotionally and

PROFILE

that it would improve my chances of finding a job tenfold. (Little did they imagine that I would go on to capitalize on my fat and become a successful actor in part as a result of it!)

Even though I felt incredible resentment at the time, I feared that I might lose my opportunity to get a master's degree from the very prestigious university I was attending. And so I—someone who had never been into drugs—started taking speed as a way to lose weight. I became addicted to illegal amphetamines—crystal meth. I snorted it and it almost ruined my nose, and when I couldn't snort it anymore, I ingested it. I did it not for the high but to lose weight, to be accepted by my peers and the faculty, and to avoid getting kicked out of school. For a food addict like myself, it made sense to me at the time. I'd been on diets that didn't work. I'd been given ultimatums by my family. I had struggled with my weight for 13 years. I saw no other alternative.

The speed was successful. I lost 80 pounds. I got down to about 175 pounds, the lowest I had ever weighed in my adult life. But that weight on my 5'10" body made me look emaciated. Still, I was celebrated by everyone—my peers and the faculty. It's fascinating. No one said, "Camryn, you certainly lost a lot of weight in a short time," or "We're concerned about you—you don't look healthy." No! They all said, "You look great! How did you do it?" I got all this praise, and I was so afraid I'd gain it back that I just kept using the amphetamines—till the day soon after graduation when I overdosed.

That's when I entered a substance-withdrawal program, plus a smoking-cessation program—I had been a smoker for 12 years, and I quit smoking at the same time. I was suicidal. There I was, quitting drugs, quitting smoking, getting out of college, and trying to enter a profession that was cruel and unforgiving. It was a very hard time.

I saw that I wasn't really ready for the acting thing, so for the

PROFILE

next two years, I devoted myself to learning sign language. I honed my skills as an interpreter for the deaf, and I became very involved with the deaf community and deaf theater. Since I had lost my weight in a very artificial way, with no behavior modification, I didn't learn anything about how to eat properly. Once off drugs, I gained all the weight back, and more. But in spite of that, I was becoming successful—I started getting kudos for my work with the deaf. I grew more confident, and my I'll-show-you! drive came back.

That's when I decided to attack my career. I became very active. I started going on auditions, as well as writing and producing my own shows, including one called *Wake Up, I'm Fat!* I was the underdog, and I started climbing the ladder one rung at a time. Now, six years later, I'm at the top! I had four movies out last year, including *The Eraser* with Arnold Schwarzenegger. I'm about to start another movie for Disney, I'm in the new David Kelley series *The Practice*, and I've had several offers from major studios to do a television series based on my character in *Wake Up, I'm Fat!* In addition, I teach acting and career development at my alma mater—and, believe me, I do everything I can to counteract the ideas I was taught there about having to be thin.

These days, I feel great. I've cut fat out of my diet because I want to have more energy. When you're on the set 14 or 15 hours a day, you have to be just as alert the fifteenth hour as you are the first, and when I'm eating a lot of fat, I tend to be more tired. And I exercise. I especially love to play competitive sports, like racquetball, and I do NordicTrack even though it's a big bore—there's nobody to beat! When I'm in New York, I try to exercise three times a week.

By exercising and eating a low-fat diet, I can maintain my weight. In fact, I've lost 30 pounds. But I'm a big woman, and I will probably always be a big woman; that's a given. While I

PROFILE

don't *love* being fat and never will, I *do* love a lot of other things about myself, and I'm no longer going to beat myself up on account of just one part of who I am.

Of course, it isn't easy. Every day we fat people are bombarded with images on bus-stop shelters, in magazines, and on commercials that tell us our bodies are unacceptable and undesirable. Trying to deal with those messages can be a lifetime struggle. Fat people are one of the last minorities who are openly and legally discriminated against without apology. America is disgusted by its overweight population. Our country is offended and embarrassed by us—and what's so ironic is that more than one-third of us are overweight! But we have to learn how not to be ashamed that we're fat and to demand the equal rights in every aspect of our life that we deserve. In all of the work I do in Hollywood, in the theater, and in my advocacy, I will try to dispel the myth that fat people aren't beautiful and desirable, because we are.

Chapter Ten

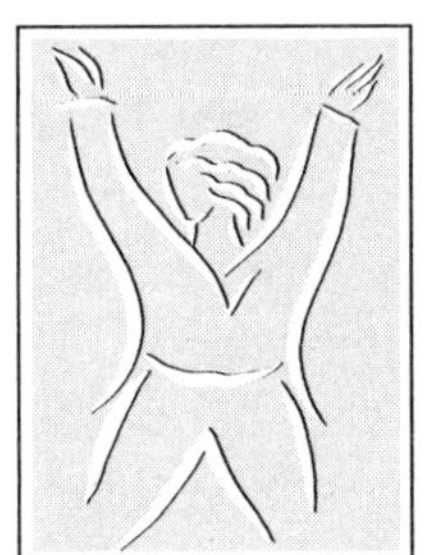

Seeing the Big Picture

Congratulations, you made it! Made *what?*, you may be thinking. After all, if this had been a diet book and you had taken its advice, you might be a little thinner by now. But, of course, this *isn't* a diet book, and there was no prescription here for weight loss. Chances are, if you hopped on the bathroom scale today, you'd probably weigh just about what you weighed when you first opened this book.

But—and it's an important but—you may be feeling like a brand-new person now that you've reached the final chapter of *Just the Weigh You Are.* That's because we've urged you to put your weight issues aside and encouraged you to think about improving your health and well-being and then *act* on those positive thoughts—to eat better, to exercise regularly, to get that stress under control, to kick the smoking habit for good. And if you've heeded our advice at all, you may already feel a whole lot better than you did on page 1—more energetic, less stressed-out, perhaps sleeping better, and just enjoying your life more.

If you've made conscious changes in your food program and

have worked to cut some of the fat from your meals, you may have discovered to your delight a newfound appreciation for simply prepared, healthy foods. It's very possible that you no longer miss those greasy fries and high-fat desserts that may have been staples of your diet. Indeed, when you do have that occasional high-fat food these days, it may actually taste *too* fatty and leave you with a case of heartburn or an upset stomach.

By now you may have also found that skipping a day or two of your exercise program leaves you feeling a bit sluggish or out of sorts—you *need* that session on your treadmill or PaceWalking through the park to get your blood pumping and your energy level soaring. And if you've succeeded in kicking the smoking habit, you may be feeling terrific, minus the cough and nicotine cravings that once plagued you. Being in the presence of smokers now, you may be finding, doesn't make you want to light up but rather to leave the room. What's more, if you were to get a checkup at the doctor's, he or she might have additional good news for you in the form of lower cholesterol, triglyceride, and blood-pressure readings.

So if you've taken some or all of these steps to help create a new-and-improved you, by all means take a well-earned bow!

Losing Weight Is Okay Too

OUR MESSAGE THROUGHOUT THIS BOOK has been clear: that you need not be thin or weigh a particular number of pounds in order to be healthy. Which is why, during all our discussion of regular exercise, low-fat eating, stress management, and other health-maintenance regimes, we deliberately played down the effect these behaviors might have on your weight. That's because, as we all know, not everyone can lose weight using traditional weight-loss methods.

But maybe—just maybe—we described a program that was new for you. Maybe you were never a regular exerciser, and suddenly you've discovered the joy of working out on a daily or almost-daily basis. Or maybe you *thought* you were eating healthfully and then began to realize that your daily fat-gram intake was really up in the stratosphere, and now, having switched to a lower-fat regime, you're liking the tastes and textures of delicious low-fat foods. And maybe the last time you happened to get on your bathroom scale, you discovered that, as a result of these positive changes in behavior, you had actually *lost* weight.

What do you know about that!

Well, we certainly didn't promise it would happen; we didn't even predict it. But it's quite possible that your new, healthier routine has induced your body to give up some fat. Great! Enjoy it, and using the weight-maintenance techniques we've talked about in this book, you might wish to try to keep that new, lower weight stable as long as you comfortably can. Recent studies have shown that even a small weight loss—as little as 7 or 10 percent of your body weight—can, in some people, produce dramatic improvements in blood pressure, blood-cholesterol levels, and diabetes management. So if these have been the outcomes for you, we're very glad.

Self-Assessment Checklist

As you know, we've been strenuously opposed to having you do a lot of heavy-duty calorie counting, regimented exercise, or list keeping. We believe that getting and staying healthy shouldn't be like doing *work.* More than anything else, improving your health status is a matter of taking control and then making simple, smart choices every day—and *continuing* to make them, for life.

But how do you know when you might not be moving forward on the path you've designed for yourself, at the pace you've chosen for yourself? And once that happens, how do you get yourself up to speed again? Periodically reviewing your health goals and reminding yourself why they're important is a very effective way to get yourself back on track. We all need a little motivational boost every now and then, and this remobilization of your motivation can take place whenever you like.

Answering the 15 questions in the checklist, below, can be quite helpful in this regard. You can make copies of the list and go over it as often as you feel the need—monthly, say, or every three months, to give you a timely review of your progress.

	YES	USUALLY	OOPS!
I review my list of long-term health goals regularly.	☐	☐	☐
I meet my weekly exercise goal.	☐	☐	☐
I weigh myself periodically to make sure I'm not gaining any significant amount of weight, and deal with it right away if I have.	☐	☐	☐
I eat a good breakfast every morning.	☐	☐	☐
I generally stick to low-fat foods.	☐	☐	☐
I eat at least five servings of fruits and vegetables a day.	☐	☐	☐
I keep the kitchen as fat-free as possible.	☐	☐	☐
I do stress-management exercises (such as progressive relaxation) when I need them.	☐	☐	☐
I drink six to eight glasses of water a day.	☐	☐	☐

	Yes	Usually	Oops!
I have exercise alternatives ready when the weather is bad and I can't exercise outdoors.	☐	☐	☐
If I feel myself backsliding with a particular behavior I'm working to change (smoking, letting stress make me frantic, etc.), I reread the appropriate chapter(s) in this book for help.	☐	☐	☐
When I need it, I seek support from others for making the lifestyle changes I'm trying to make.	☐	☐	☐
I reward myself whenever I reach one of my interim goals.	☐	☐	☐

If you don't see as many Yes or Usually answers as you'd like to, don't despair. Focus on the areas where you responded Oops! and see if you can't do better the next time you review the list.

The Joy of Eating

We're hoping that one of the benefits you derive from having read this book is a brand-new appreciation for food.

No, we're not kidding.

We realize that eating may have been an emotionally charged issue for you in the past and that the love-hate relationship so many overweight people have with food may make it impossible to view it objectively or positively. But we sincerely hope that by focusing not on your weight but on healthy eating and other good habits, you'll come to realize—as do many people who have never had a weight problem—that food is indeed one of the joys of living.

Yes, we've stressed low-fat eating throughout this book, and we're certainly not backing down on its importance now. But we're all human, regardless of our size, and there are few of us who don't have *one* fat-packed favorite, whether it's chocolate-chocolate-chip ice cream, pepperoni pizza, or highly marbled sirloin steak. Everyone is entitled to a rare fat-be-damned treat, particularly when it marks a significant event. That slice of cake at your daughter's wedding, that celebratory glass of spiked eggnog to welcome in the New Year—even that hot dog and beer on a glorious summer day at the ballpark—are wonderful opportunities that should not be missed. None of these isolated high-fat culinary events *made* you overweight, and they're not going to make you heavier or put you at greater risk for disease *if* you keep them infrequent, limited in size—and if you appreciate them when they occur.

We all know that some foods are better for our overall health than others, and those are the ones that should have starring roles in your food plan. But *no* food is or should be completely off-limits. Do keep an eye on your health and your present weight range, but *don't* become a killjoy who refuses to let some delicious piece of food pass his or her lips because of some rigid, self-imposed rule. Life's too short for such needless sacrifices.

Give Yourself a Break

In the beginning of a brand-new program—when you're really motivated to do everything you're supposed to do to get healthy—it's almost impossible to keep your enthusiasm and motivation down. You actually catch yourself thinking things like, Hey, why haven't I ever noticed how *good* cauliflower tastes? or I'm going to finish my run. It isn't raining *that* hard.

Yes, those are the golden days of any wellness program. But the best-laid plans . . . We don't mean to be negative, merely realistic. The fact is, it's tough to exercise five times a week when you've got the flu. It's difficult to get freshly steamed vegetables when you're on vacation in Mexico. And it's a challenge to keep your stress level down when the house painters are entering their third week on the job.

Sooner or later, Real Life is going to intrude on your new, healthy, well-managed lifestyle, and keeping it up won't be as easy. Just do the best you can, and give yourself permission to ease up on yourself and your program when it's absolutely necessary. What separates the healthy men from the boys and the healthy women from the girls is knowing the importance of getting back on track as soon as you are able—not letting too much time go by before you get back into the exercise and healthy-eating groove, managing your stress and your personal safety—whatever may have temporarily gone by the boards.

Living in the Real World

TEMPORARY DEVIATION from your healthy program is one thing; abandoning it is quite another.

We've talked throughout this book about the importance of keeping your motivation mobilized so that you can continue moving forward toward your health goals and maintain them once you achieve them. And we strongly urge you to return to Chapter Four whenever you sense that what's-the-point-of-it-all feeling creep over you and you know that your commitment needs a boost.

But there's a different kind of scenario, apart from sluggish motivation, that may gradually bring down all your hard work to date. We're talking about those high-risk and unexpected situations, those life events that shake up our well-ordered routines and tempt us to slip back into those old, unfortunate patterns that caused us to lead less-than-healthy lives to begin with. No one is immune. We all encounter those situations—whether it's a prolonged illness that keeps us from our exercise routine, or the loss of a job, or a personal tragedy that sends our emotions soaring and makes getting our five daily servings of fruits and vegetables seem like the most trivial thing in the world.

But, as you know, we've been urging you all along to keep your eye on the Big Picture that is your life, to decide what's important and what's unimportant, and to make the commitment to yourself to change your lifestyle for the better for the sake of your health and longevity. And that means not throwing in the towel on your healthy-living program when something major comes along (as it inevitably will) to disrupt your day-to-day routine. It's time—perhaps for the first time in your life—to put achieving wellness and maintaining your peace of mind right at the top of your personal agenda. This may mean balancing your obligations to other duties and other people with your obligations to yourself. That may be difficult for you to do, but at certain times in your life, your health and well-being may depend on it.

Sometimes, the strength of our commitment to ourselves really gets tested. For example, we know a woman who, after years of on-and-off attempts to stick to a program of regular exercise and healthy eating, had finally gotten her act together. She joined a gym and was going several times a week. She had found, to her delight, that after several months, she actually enjoyed walking on the treadmill and lifting weights, and she was proud of the muscles and the toned body she was developing at the age of 44. Coupled with her newfound enthusiasm for regular exercise was a fresh appreciation for healthy eating—good, flavorful, highly seasoned dishes that were low in fat and nutritionally sound. Formerly a smoker, she hadn't picked up a cigarette in 18 months.

Then, her healthy, well-organized life took an unfortunate turn. Her 73-year-old widowed mother developed cancer, and her prognosis wasn't good. Suddenly, the daughter found herself spending days and nights in a hospital, tending to her mother's needs and worrying constantly about her condition. In the past, it was situations like this—far less stressful ones, in fact—that would send the daughter into an eating and cigarette-smoking frenzy. When her mother died, the daughter's pain was almost overwhelming. But she also thought about how far she had come with her healthier lifestyle and how proud of her her mother had been. And, the daughter had to admit to herself, No amount of bingeing on ice cream or smoking cigarettes is going to bring my mother back.

So throughout the pain and emotional stress of the days and weeks that followed, the woman remained faithful to her health program. She even found that it gave her strength, physically, of course, but also psychologically, to know she hadn't let herself fall apart during what was conceivably the most difficult time in her life. She could have easily gone back to her old bad habits, and no one would have blamed or criticized her. But she was now past the point of allowing events and stresses to rule her life. She was in charge—and it felt very good.

It's crucial that we all figure out ahead of time how we're going to handle the next curveball that life throws us—without abandoning our commitment to live a healthy, happy life in the body we're in. Here are some strategies for dealing sensibly with stressful events and high-risk situations:

• **Rest more.** Give yourself more "space," more time to be alone (if that's what you feel you need), to sleep more at night or take daytime naps, to go for a walk in the middle of the day when your emotions or stress levels threaten to get the best of you.

• **Talk it out.** Talk to a trusted friend, relative, or therapist. Find a person who can give you the time and emotional support you need and can be as judgment-free as possible.

• **Write it down.** When things seem too much to handle, jot down your feelings. Just the act of putting on paper a description of your emotional responses and what's causing them will make them more manageable.

• **Develop your assertiveness skills.** The real-life profiles you've been reading throughout this book are full of insightful ways overweight women and men have learned to stand up to the saboteurs and naysayers in their lives. The negative people in your life may range from ones who urge you to eat that fattening dessert when you don't want it to people whose eyes burn holes through the groceries in your shopping cart to those who insist you'll never be truly healthy unless you weigh 135 pounds.

Assertiveness doesn't come easily for many of us, but it may be crucial if you finally want to be at peace with yourself and your weight. Speaking up (and directly) works well for some large-size people and in some situations; for others, ignoring that look or comment may be the best bet. Asking for help and support ("Honey, please come with me for a walk after dinner tonight.") can be surprisingly effective. And if all else fails, you may simply find that that person who can't or won't understand you and your feelings no longer deserves a place in your life.

• **Plan what you can.** It's far easier to stay in charge of our healthy routine when we anticipate problems. Let's say you must visit relatives who always upset you (and tend to send you sliding into bad health habits). Figure out how you can fulfill your social obligation without the typical aftermath. Some suggestions: cut your usual visiting time in half; bring along an amusing friend to lighten the atmosphere; eat a healthy snack before you leave your house so you're not tempted to eat inappropriately during the visit; practice deep-breathing exercises before, during, and after the get-together to keep you calm.

• **Stick to your healthy program as closely as possible.** Give yourself credit for being able to weather the storms without blowing your program. If you're not as successful now as you usually are in terms of staying active and eating sensibly, just do the best you can without giving up altogether. Once things settle down, you'll find it easier to pick up where you left off if you haven't quit your program completely.

• **Remind yourself why you're doing all this.** Yes, this may be a time of high stress, depression, or frustration. But don't lose sight of how far you've come. You've just devoted the last few weeks or months of your life to a program designed to improve your health, your longevity, your self-esteem, and your happiness. Aren't these things important enough to work at and hold onto forever?

Self-Acceptance

OPEN ANY POPULAR DIET BOOK and you're sure to see most of the same elements you've seen in weight-loss books all your life: an eating plan, perhaps a list of low-fat foods, a recommendation to do some exercise, and a clear-cut message about how much healthier and happier you'll be when you finally drop those 50 or 75 pounds.

But if you've stayed with us throughout these pages of *Just the Weigh You Are*, you're bound to look with justified skepticism at any diet book's predictions for your health and happiness. You've been there, you've done that, and no guru's weight-loss formula has ever worked long-term for you. Even more importantly, you know by now that health is not accurately rated simply by the numbers on your scale. You're aware now that you can take control of your health by taking control of other areas of your life—via regular exercise, nutritious eating, smoking cessation, and the like. You may not be focusing on getting thinner as a result of these activities, but for a variety of other reasons, you'll feel great once they've become a permanent part of your life.

Which brings us to the subject of self-acceptance, of finally coming to terms with who you are, knowing what's important for *you*, and feeling okay about the body you're presently in. Sadly, despite our wish to the contrary, we live in a world that can be quite unforgiving; any deviation from the norm (whatever "the norm" is) is regarded with scorn or mockery. And even though about one-third of the American population today is overweight, that still leaves plenty of others who may look with contempt and feelings of superiority at those of us who can't slip into a size 10 and never will.

Yes, it takes grit and self-esteem to say, firmly and self-confidently, "I think I'm fine just the way I am. I may not be model-thin, but I don't need that to be happy, healthy, or feel good about myself." If you can make such a statement and really *believe* it in your heart—without thinking in the back of your mind that come Monday or New Year's Day, you just *might* give those new diet pills a whirl—then you deserve tremendous respect and admiration.

Because you still live in a society that has a long way to go toward accepting variety and difference, and you've chosen to go your own individual way.

Nevertheless, your positive attitude and determination notwithstanding, you have to realize that you're going to find yourself coming face-to-face with people of all shapes and sizes who will *never* accept themselves the way they are (and will expect you to feel the same). There will be people who count the number of peas on their plate and who exercise for hours at a time in the hopes of moving their belts one notch in. You're going to find yourself in the company of folks who compliment one another on how skinny they've become, and when they get around to noticing you, they'll quickly change the subject. There may still be those times in your life—at the pool, in the dressing room, when disrobing for a new lover—when you'll feel a twinge (or two) of insecurity about your body.

The question is, Can you live with all that? We sincerely hope so, because if you can't, you'll continually drive yourself crazy and may possibly do damage to your health in your quest for slimness. But if you *can* accept yourself and your weight as they are, then something wonderful will happen. You'll be discovering a new serenity, an unexpected peacefulness within you that you never knew existed. You'll finally be able to get on with your life, focus on the Big Picture we've been talking about, and figure out what really matters to you. Without fixating on your weight anymore, you'll find that your mind is clearer than ever and that you've suddenly inherited more time and energy than you ever thought possible.

In short, you'll have a big weight off you.

If you do choose this route, we applaud you, and we urge you to remain sensible even as you turn your back on your weight obsessions of the past. Eat what you like, but use good common sense when you do. Exercise regularly for all the health benefits *and* all the psychological rewards you will reap. Keep that stress under control with the techniques we've provided for you in these pages. And periodically review the relevant chapters in this book whenever you feel your commitment to your health slowly start to slip away.

Just like the strong, self-confident, large-size women and men whose stories appear in these pages, learn to trust yourself and your own instincts. You're smarter and tougher than you think. For deciding to live in the body you have—but with the goal of making it healthier—congratulate yourself for giving yourself a well-deserved break, and for having the wisdom and courage to follow your head instead of the herd.

PROFILE

Juanita Harvey

Brooklyn, New York
Age: 40
Height: 5'2"
Weight: 212 pounds
Occupation: Executive director of a nonprofit organization

I COME FROM A FAMILY OF HEAVY WOMEN, but I was always one of the thinner ones. Until my late 20s, I weighed 110 pounds. Then, I had surgery in 1987—I had a ruptured cyst, and an ovary and a fallopian tube were removed. I was in a great deal of pain and incapacitated for about three months; I was also eating more and drinking a lot of beer. So I put on weight, and I've been overweight ever since. Over the last eight years, I've been as much as 230, although I'm comfortable now weighing between 205 and 210.

When I put on weight, it didn't come as a shock—that was what was supposed to happen if you ate more and weren't active, and I had been fairly active before then. I tried to lose weight with different diets and diet products—Ultra Slim-Fast, a high-protein diet, and one or two others—but I never stayed with any of them for long. So then my weight just became a matter of my accepting it, which I did. I knew I still wanted to be active—in fact, I got involved with wrestling four years ago because, unlike something like tennis where you have to do a lot of running, weight is not an obstacle in wrestling. So it was ideal for me.

After I gained weight, I also started to think about how my weight might be an advantage to me in other ways. As I said,

PROFILE

the women in my family were heavy—one grandmother weighed about 250 pounds, the other one was also heavy, and my mother weighs 200 and change. They're also all strong and independent—for example, my mother raised five kids pretty much by herself. So I started equating weight with strength and power. I had positive role models among the heavy (and good-looking) women in my family. To my mind, being heavy wasn't a matter of being ugly or having a negative body image—it meant strength and substance.

My attitude about my weight comes not only from having strong role models in my family but also from accepting my culture. In some African tribes, having a physically substantial woman meant a man was rich. I relate to that idea. Although there's still the negative image of the African-American women in the South who were the mammies and the cooks, the fact is they were the ones who managed those families. There's a lot of strength associated with being heavy, a lot that is nourishing to others.

I know we live in a world where people are often judged by their weight, and in my psychotherapy sessions, I've discussed my weight a lot. At one point, I needed to look for a job, and I was concerned about my prospects because I didn't have a so-called "front-office appearance"—that was something I talked about in therapy. But eventually I did get a job I like, and today I don't worry about how others may react to my appearance, on the job or off. In my mind, I'm a good person and I'm positive about myself, and that will be reflected to those open to it. If people allow my appearance to affect their opinion of me, that's their hang-up.

As far as I'm concerned, I'm fine. My weight doesn't hold me back. I can run upstairs like everyone else—there's no elevator in the building where I live, so I go up and down the stairs several times a day. Five days a week, I carry a bag that

PROFILE

weighs 20 or 25 pounds to and from work, so I have a lot of definition in my shoulders, back, and arms from carrying it. Four days a week, I do stretching exercises, and on Saturdays, I play softball. And before the annual Gay Games, I train every day for a couple of months. [*Editor's note:* Juanita won a gold medal in wrestling in the 1994 Gay Games in New York City.]

As for food, I don't usually overeat, but at the same time, I'm not afraid of tiramisu or chocolate mousse—when I want something, I'll have it.

I believe that, to be valued, you have to have an idea of your value—and it's not your weight that's keeping you from having value. If there are issues, address them. If something is keeping you from appreciating yourself, find out what that thing is. What's tragic is that we as a society are losing the contributions of so many wonderful people who have gone into hiding just because they think they're not skinny enough.

PROFILE

Pat Miller

Westmont, Illinois
Age: 42
Height: 5'2"
Weight: 220 pounds
Occupation: Homemaker (currently)

I BEGAN HAVING WEIGHT PROBLEMS as an adolescent. I had asthma, and because of that, I was kept out of physical education programs, so I was pretty inactive. Also, whenever I had any discretionary money, I would spend it on sweets. My brother and I used to love eating graham crackers with frosting on them.

Before I started high school, I was put on a doctor's diet. It was very low-calorie and very restrictive in terms of what I could eat. I lost 80 pounds, bringing my weight down to about 135. I stayed below 160 pounds throughout high school. In college, I discovered physical education again, and I was very active, but my weight fluctuated a lot, and I eventually went up to 180 pounds.

After graduation, I got a job as an international tour guide. For eight years, I traveled the world, and I enjoyed it very much. For several years after that, I worked in corporate travel. My weight was definitely an issue in getting hired. It was never said, of course, but finding me the right-size uniform became an issue, so I just had mine custom-made. None of this bothered me—I was so oblivious to the bosses' reactions to my weight. After all, I was in my dream job; it was something I had always wanted since I was young child. In fact, I've always done what I've really wanted to do. I haven't let people say no to me. It took me four years to get that first tour-guide job, but

PROFILE

because it was my dream, I tried not to let anything stand in the way of my getting it. Part of it was luck, but part of it was determination.

I made the official decision to stop dieting during the last 3 years, but I really haven't dieted seriously in the last 10. I was never a big dieter. I've actually only been on two serious diets—the one before high school and the one before my wedding in 1985, when I went on Optifast and lost 50 or 60 pounds. Of course, the weight all came back, and more. Going up and down, I probably did a lot of harm to my health at the time, so that was it for me in terms of dieting.

These days, I try to eat healthfully, but I eat whatever I want. If I want something healthy, I'll eat it, and if I want something fattening, I'll eat that. But I don't binge. Food used to be a source of anxiety for me, but not anymore.

I'm also very physically active. I've been a volunteer teaching fitness classes at the local Y, and I taught aqua aerobics up until the ninth month of my pregnancy. In the summer, my daughter and I swim at the community swimming pool every day, and two days a week, I walk for exercise. During the other months, I usually swim a couple of days a week, work out with weights one or two days a week at the Y, and exercise at home with a personal trainer once a week.

I'd say my health is good—no high blood pressure, no diabetes, none of the illnesses usually associated with overweight. I get regular health checkups. Besides the asthma I've had all my life, I've also had arthritis since I was a teenager. It's starting to be more painful, but I'm getting into my 40s, so maybe it's an age thing. But I definitely see a correlation between my exercise routine and my arthritis: If I don't do a certain amount of exercise every week, my arthritis is worse. Exercise keeps it from getting *too* painful, though.

Unlike a lot of large-size people, I was never miserable about

PROFILE

my weight, and throughout my life, I didn't alter my behavior because of it. I'm certainly aware of the cultural norm about weight, but I'd say that anything I did in terms of dieting was a reaction to comments from my mother (she's obsessed about my weight and always has been) or other people, rather than something *I* wanted to do. For example, when I started working out with my personal trainer last year, the issue of weight came up. I told her I was working out to become more fit, and if I lost weight, great, but it wasn't my goal—my goal was to be as fit as I could be. In fact, I don't think I've lost any weight with the trainer, but I'm definitely stronger and feeling better.

I was recently thinking back over my life, especially about the time when I was a tour guide and in contact with so many people. I realized that I was more accepting of myself and my body than my thinner counterparts were of themselves and their bodies. I knew this because it would come up in conversation. For example, as far as how people looked in bathing suits, others were always much more self-conscious about that than I was. Why? I suppose it's something at my core. As I've said, I was pretty accepting of myself all through life, even as a child. What was hard was everyone else's comments, especially in childhood—children are so cruel. As you reach adulthood, there are fewer comments, but even then, whenever I heard them, I could deal with them. The hard part is dealing with other people who can't accept my body.

I think there's still a great deal of prejudice in this country against big people. I'm not an activist; I don't do anything about this issue in an organized fashion. But I feel that, as a big person, if I can convince just one person a day that I'm okay, that's good.

Resources

Publications, organizations, and services of particular interest to large-size women and men

Books

Atrens, Dale. *Don't Diet.* William Morrow, 1988.

Bennett, William & Gurin, Joel. *The Dieter's Dilemma.* HarperCollins, 1983.

Chernin, Kim. *The Hungry Self.* HarperCollins, 1986.

Chernin, Kim. *The Obsession: Reflections on the Tyranny of Slenderness.* Harper & Row, 1981.

Cooke, Kaz. *Real Gorgeous: The Truth About Body & Beauty.* Norton, 1996.

Curtis, Lucy D.L. *Lucy's List: A Comprehensive Sourcebook for Making Larger Living Easier.* Warner, 1995.

Dixon, Monica, M.S., R.D. *Love the Body You Were Born With: A Ten-Step Workbook for Women.* Perigee, 1996.

Erdman, Cheri K. *Nothing to Lose: A Guide to Sane Living in a Larger Body.* HarperCollins, 1995.

Farro, Rita. *Life Is Not a Dress Size.* Chilton, 1996.

Foreyt, John & Goodrick, G. Ken. *Living Without Dieting.* Warner Books, 1992.

Garrison, Terry. *Fed-Up! A Woman's Guide to Freedom from the Diet/Weight Prison.* Carroll & Graf, 1993.

Goodman, W. Charisse. *The Invisible Woman: Confronting Weight Prejudice in America.* Gurze, 1995.

Hall, Lindsey. *Full Lives: Women Who Have Freed Themselves from Food and Weight Obsession.* Gurze, 1993.

Healthy Weight Journal, eds. *Afraid to Eat: Children and Teens in Weight Crisis.* (Available for $21.95 from *Healthy Weight Journal*, 402 S. 14th Street, Hettinger, ND 58639.)

Healthy Weight Journal, eds. *The Health Risks of Weight Loss.* (Available for $21.95 from *Healthy Weight Journal*, 402 S. 14th Street, Hettinger, ND 58639.)

Higgs, Liz Curtis. *One Size Fits All and Other Fables.* Thomas Nelson, 1993.

Hirschmann, Jane & Munter, Carol. *Overcoming Overeating.* Fawcett, 1988.

Hirschmann, Jane & Munter, Carol. *When Women Stop Hating Their Bodies.* Fawcett, 1995.

Hollis, Judy, Ph.D. *Fat and Furious.* Ballantine, 1994.

Johnson, Carol A. *Self-Esteem Comes in All Sizes.* Doubleday, 1996.

Jonas, Steven, M.D. *Take Control of Your Weight.* Consumer Reports Books, 1993.

Kano, Susan. *Making Peace with Food.* Harper & Row, 1989.

Lakein, Alan. *How To Get Control of Your Time and Life.* Penguin, 1974.

Lyons, Pat & Burgard, Debora. *Great Shape: The First Fitness Guide for Large Women.* Bull Publishing, 1988.

Mayer, Ken. *Real Women Don't Diet!* Pinnacle, 1993.

NAAFA (National Association to Advance Fat Acceptance). *The NAAFA Workbook: A Complete Study Guide.* NAAFA, 1987.

Newman, Leslea. *Some Body to Love: A Guide to Loving the Body You Have.* K Side Press, 1991.

Northrup, Christine. *Women's Bodies, Women's Wisdom: Creating Physical and Emotional Health and Healing.* Bantam, 1994.

Omichinski, Linda, R.D. *You Count, Calories Don't: The Hugs™ Plan for Better Health.* Tamos Books, (800) 565-4847.

Orbach, Susie. *Fat Is a Feminist Issue.* Berkeley, 1990.

Ray, Sondra. *The Only Diet There Is.* Celestial Arts, 1981.

Roberts, Nancy. *Breaking All the Rules: Feeling Good and Looking Great No Matter What Your Size.* Penguin, 1985.

Rodin, Judith. *Body Traps.* Quill/William Morrow, 1992.

Roth, Geneen. *When Food Is Love.* Plume, 1991.

Schroeder, Charles Roy, Ph.D. *Fat Is Not a Four-Letter Word.* Chronimed Publishing, 1992.

Seid, Roberta P. *Never Too Thin: Why Women Are at War with Their Bodies.* Prentice-Hall, 1989.

Schwartz, Hillel. *Never Satisfied: A Cultural History of Diets, Fantasies and Fat.* The Free Press, 1986.

Stacey, Michelle. *Consumed: Why Americans Love, Hate and Fear Food.* Simon & Schuster, 1994.

Winston, Stephanie. *Getting Organized.* Warner, 1991.

Wolf, Naomi. *The Beauty Myth: How Images of Beauty are Used Against Women.* Anchor, 1992.

Other References

The Eating Disorders Bookshelf Catalog
Gurze Books
P.O. Box 2238
Carlsbad, CA 92018
(800) 756-7533
http://www.gurze.com (web site)
Features more than 100 books and tapes dealing with eating disorders, body image, size acceptance, and self-esteem.

BodyTrust video (produced by Ms. Dale Hayes, R.D.)
2110 Overland Avenue
Suite 120
Billings, MT 59102
(800) 321-9499
This 60-minute video (for $28.95) deals with "undieting" your way to health and happiness.

The Food Guide Pyramid: Your Personal Guide to Healthful Eating
For a free copy, send a self-addressed, stamped, business-size envelope to:
The International Food Information Council Foundation
1100 Connecticut Avenue NW
Suite 430
Washington, DC 20036
(202) 296-6540

Nutrition and Your Health: Dietary Guidelines for Americans
Send 50 cents per copy (check or money order, payable to Superintendent of Documents) to:
Consumer Information Center
Dept. 378-C
Pueblo, CO 81009

Magazines & Journals

Belle (a magazine for large women of color)
P.O. Box 419
Mt. Morris, IL 61054-0132
(800) 877-5549

Big Beautiful Woman (BBW)
8484 Wilshire Boulevard, #900
Beverly Hills, CA 90211
(800) 707-5592

EXTRA! (a monthly magazine for voluptuous women)
P.O. Box 57194
Sherman Oaks, CA 91413

Healthy Weight Journal
Healthy Living Institute
402 S. 14th Street
Hettinger, ND 58639
(701) 567-2646
(701) 567-2602 (fax)
$59 per year (six issues).

Radiance, the Magazine for Large Women
P.O. Box 30246
Oakland, CA 94604
(510) 482-0680 (phone and fax)

Rump Parliament (dedicated to size acceptance, anti-dieting and size-rights activism)
P.O. Box 181716
Dallas, TX 75218
$24 in U.S., $28 in Canada (six issues per year, sample issue $6).

Organizations

Abundia
(Programs for the Promotion of Body-Size
Acceptance and Self-Esteem)
P.O. Box 252
Downers Grove, IL 60515
(708) 897-9796
Offers a free brochure along with information on its workshops in size acceptance, self-esteem, and training for professionals who work with large-size people.

AHELP (Association for the Health
Enrichment of Large Persons)
Dr. Joseph McVoy, Director
P.O. Box 11743
Blacksburg, VA 24062
(540) 951-3527
AHELP@nrv.net (e-mail)
AHELP's mission is to educate people about the dangers of dieting and to give alternatives to dieting; offers referrals to health and psychological professionals supportive of large-size people. Call, write, or e-mail for an information packet.

Ample Opportunity
P.O. Box 40621
Portland, OR 97240
(503) 245-1524
Promotes health, well-being, and size acceptance for women.

Body Image Task Force
P.O. Box 934
Santa Cruz, CA 95061
Their goal is to fight size discrimination and lookism, and to promote a positive body image for all people. Four free brochures available (send three 32-cent stamps).

Council on Size & Weight Discrimination
(includes the International No Diet Day Coalition)
P.O. Box 305
Mt. Marion, NY 12456
(914) 679-1209
(914) 679-1206 (fax)
Offers a free brochure and a comprehensive bibliography of books on body image, health, and size acceptance.

Diet/Weight Liberation
Terry Nicholetti Garrison, Director
c/o Anabel Taylor Hall
Cornell University
Ithaca, NY 14853
Send a stamped, self-addressed envelope to receive information on how you can promote weight-acceptance/weight-liberation activities in your area.

HUGS™ International (nondiet lifestyle program)
Box 102A, R.R. #3
Portage la Prairie, Manitoba
Canada R1N 3A3
(204) 428-3432
(800) 565-4847 (for ordering information)
(204) 428-5072 (fax)
lomichin@portage.net (e-mail)
http://www.hugs.com (web site)
Send a stamped, self-addressed envelope for a listing of nondiet programs in your area, information on the HUGS™ at Home Program, and a support newsletter.

Largely Positive
P.O. Box 17223
Glendale, WI 53217
Send a stamped, self-addressed, business-size envelope for information on how to set up a support group for king-size people and for how to subscribe to the newsletter "On a Positive Note."

Largesse: Network for Size Esteem
P.O. Box 9404
New Haven, CT 06534
(203) 787-1624 (phone and fax)
Send $18 for Size Empowerment kit.
NAAFA (National Association to
Advance Fat Acceptance)
P.O. Box 188620
Sacramento, CA 95818
(916) 558-6880
(916) 558-6881 (fax)
http://naafa.org (web site)
Has chapters around the country; holds convention; offers a bimonthly newsletter, pen-pal program, etc.

Index